Allergies and Children

A Handbook for Parents from The Hospital for Sick Children

Prepared by:
Dr. Milton Gold, M.D., F.R.C.P. (C)
Dr. Barry Zimmerman, M.D., F.R.C.P. (C)

With contributions from:
Dr. Gordon Donsky, M.D., F.R.C.P. (C)
Dr. Arthur Fremes, M.D., F.R.C.P. (C)
Dr. Howard Langer, M.D., F.R.C.P. (C)
Dr. Euna Lee-Hong, M.D., F.R.C.P. (C)
Dr. Riaz Nizami, M.D., F.R.C.P. (C)

Allergy Division, Department of Paediatrics,
The Hospital for Sick Children, Toronto

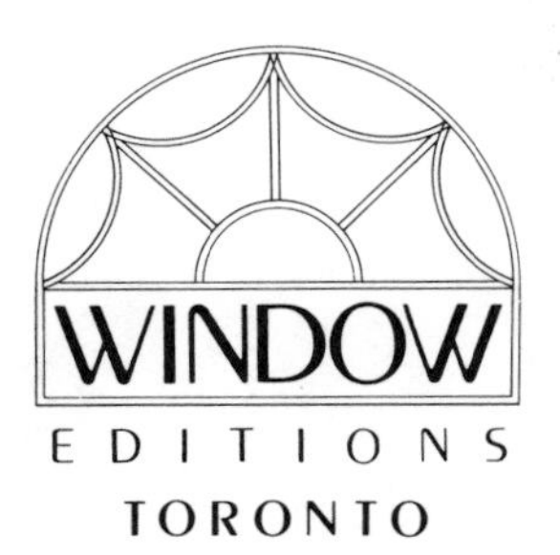

This book is dedicated to **Dr. Cecil Collins-Williams**, M.D., F.R.C.P. (C.), former Chief of the Allergy Division, Hospital for Sick Children.

Window Editions is an imprint of **Kids Can Press Ltd.**

Kids Can Press Ltd. gratefully acknowledges the assistance of the Canada Council and the Ontario Arts Council in the production of this book.

Canadian Cataloguing in Publication Data
Main entry under title:
Allergies and children: A Handbook for Parents from The Hospital for Sick Children

Includes index.
ISBN 0-919964-89-3 (pbk.)

1. Pediatric allergy — Handbooks, manuals, etc.
I. Hospital for Sick Children. Allergy Division.
RJ386.A43 1986 618.92'97 C86-093294-X

Typeset by Alphabets
Printed and bound in Canada
Edited by Valerie Wyatt
Book design by Michael Solomon
Kids Can Press Ltd., Toronto

86 0 9 8 7 6 5 4 3 2

Contents

Foreword

In the past two decades there have been significant advances in our understanding, and treatment, of allergic diseases. Management of many allergic problems is now possible without using extreme forms of treatment. Children and parents need not be frightened of their problems since they can now often control their allergies with conservative or ''middle of the road'' approaches. What is essential is education of families as to how to achieve these goals.

This book was written to respond to these needs. Originally compiled in 1983 under the supervision of the former Chief of the Allergy Division at this hospital, Dr. Cecil Collins-Williams, it was handed out to parents who brought their children into the hospital's allergy clinic. The response was gratifying, so much so that it was decided to expand and update the book and try to reach more people. Input came from many sources – from the doctors who worked on the original chapters, from Susan Daglish at the Allergy Information Association of Ontario and, again, from parents. We would like to thank all who contributed.

Of course no book can take the place of advice and suggestions from your family doctor, paediatrician or allergist. It is our hope that *Allergies and Children* will answer your questions about your child's allergies and give you tips on how to minimize his or her discomfort.

Dr. Milton Gold
June 1986
Toronto

Introduction

If you have an allergic child, you are not alone. Allergies are one of the most common long-term disorders in North America and affect 10 to 20 percent of all children.

Allergies come in many forms and degrees of severity. Your child may have unpleasant but minor nasal stuffiness or a severe case of allergy-related asthma that limits his or her activity. He or she may have a lifetime problem or one that passes with adolescence. Fortunately recent advances in the treatment of allergies mean that the vast majority of allergy sufferers, even those with severe asthma, can lead close-to-normal lives.

Your involvement can play an important role in your child's allergy problem. Using some of the suggestions outlined in *Coping with the environment*, chapter 10, you can make changes in your home that may significantly improve your child's allergy symptoms. Before you do so, however, take time to read through the chapters describing your child's allergies. Learning more about his or her problem can give you a good foundation from which to plan changes.

Raising an allergic child may be trying at times. Although most of the care falls into manageable routines, there are bound to be times of emotional strains on parents and on other non-affected children in the family. Strategies for dealing with school and emotional problems your child may experience are described at the end of this book. Your family doctor will also be able to give you specific advice on these problems.

Allergies range from uncomfortable to activity-limiting to, occasionally, life-threatening. The more you know about them and about treating them the safer and healthier your child will be.

1

Ten basic questions about allergies

1. What is an allergy?

When we say someone has an allergy, we simply mean that he or she reacts to substance(s) that do not produce harmful effects in the majority of people. These substances are called allergens. People come into contact with allergens either by breathing, eating or touching them or by having them injected into their skin or veins. The most common allergens are tree pollen, grasses and weeds, moulds, house dust, animal products such as dander (skin scales) or saliva, insect bites and stings, food and drugs.

2. How do these things cause an allergic reaction?

When a foreign substance (allergen) enters the body of an allergic child, it causes a response, which we call an allergy. Allergens prompt the body to produce proteins called antibodies. The allergen and antibody react together on the surface of "mast cells" which are found in the lining of the nose, lungs, skin and intes-

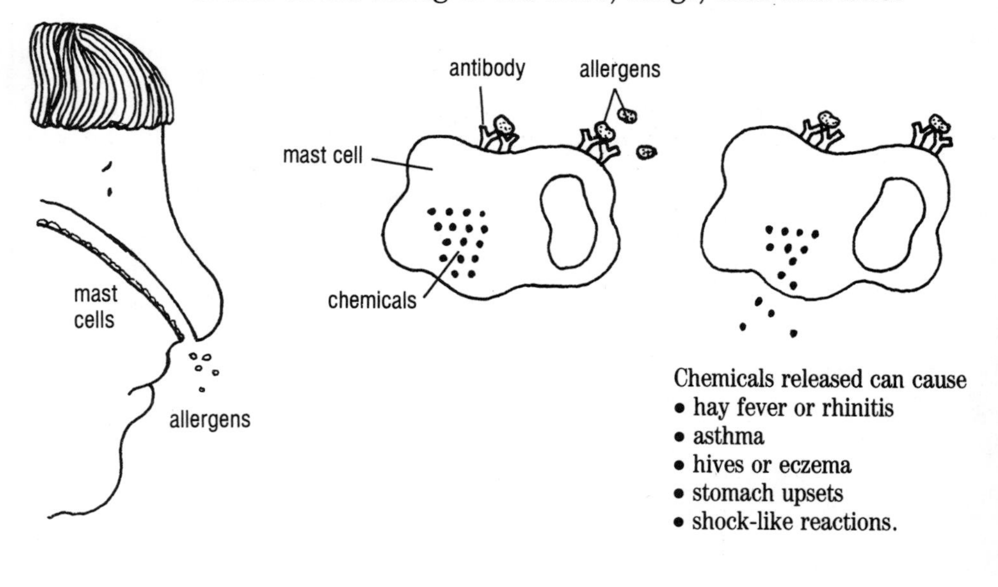

tines. The mast cells then release chemicals that cause inflammation in various parts of the body:

- in the nose there is swelling of the lining with mucus production. (This condition is called hay fever or allergic rhinitis);
- in the chest there may be swelling and mucus production in the breathing tubes (bronchi) leading to the lungs, along with spasm of these tubes (asthma);
- in the skin, inflammatory changes may develop in the form of hives or eczema;
- stomach upsets such as diarrhea, vomiting and/or bloating may be indicative of allergic reactions;
- Shock-like reactions or complete collapse (anaphylaxis) may develop as well, depending on the severity of the above reactions.

3. Who can get allergies?

Approximately 10 to 20 per cent of the population have some kind of allergy. Anyone can get allergies, regardless of age, race or sex. However, allergies are more common in young children than in adults. Asthma is found in 5 to 10 per cent of children; hay fever in 7 per cent; and 6 per cent of children have other allergic diseases such as hives, eczema, etc.

4. Are allergies inherited?

Yes – at least the tendency to develop allergies is inherited. If both you and your spouse have allergies, your child has a 60 to 75 per cent chance of developing an allergic tendency. If only one of you is allergic, then there is a 25 to 50 per cent chance, and if neither of you have allergies then there is a 10 per cent chance, similar to the rest of the population.

A child is not necessarily born with the same allergy as the parents have; the child may have asthma although the father has hay fever and the mother eczema. Also, the child's allergies can be either worse or milder than the father's or mother's.

5. Why do my allergic children become ill even when not around their allergens?

Allergies produce irritation and inflammation of various areas of the body. This leads to an increased sensitivity, or ''twitchiness,'' in these areas. Once this has happened, other factors such as cold weather, dampness, rapid weather changes, tobacco smoke, pollution and exercise may then cause further irritation. The result is similar to the reaction to an allergen.

Allergy sufferers are rarely sensitive to just one thing. They tend to be sensitive to combinations of things. So, for example, if your child is allergic to ragweed, he or she may have more problems with other irritants in ragweed season than at other times in the

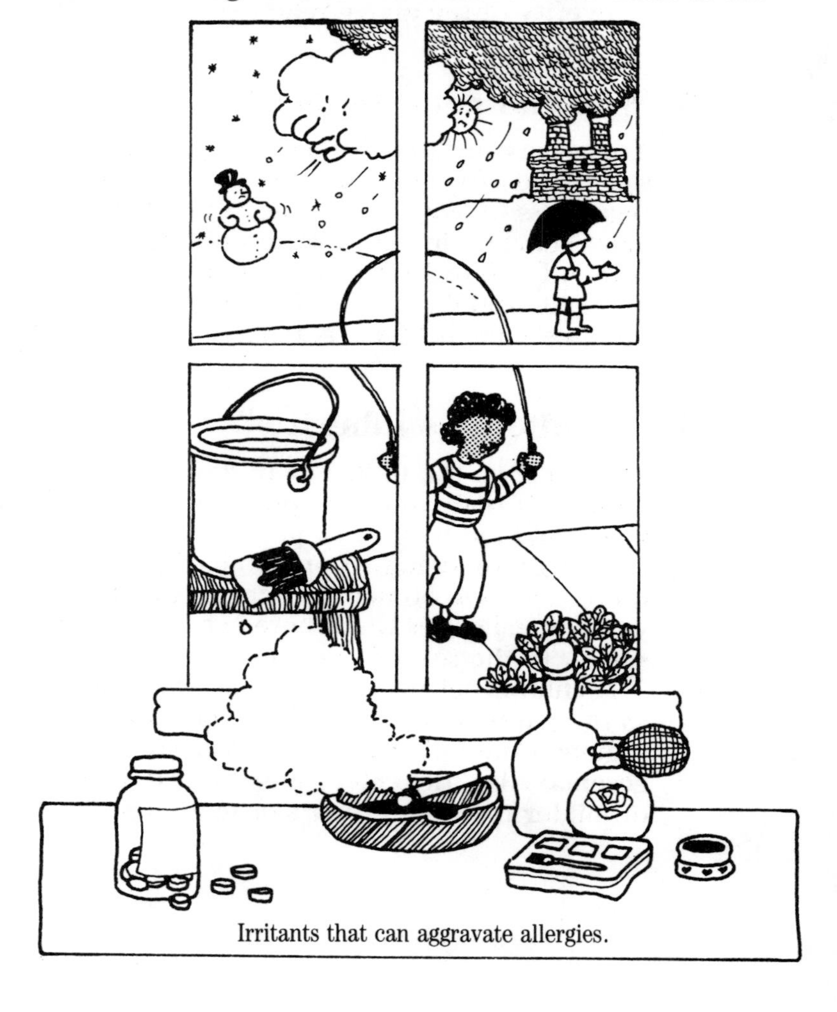

Irritants that can aggravate allergies.

year. Or if your child has a cold, allergies and/or irritants may bother him or her more at that time. Reactions to allergens are just one small part of what can affect the allergic, or ''hypersensitive,'' patient.

6. Do allergies change with time?

Yes. A child may develop some allergies early in life, while others may take years to develop. Or the pattern of your child's reactions may change over the years. For example, a sensitivity to ragweed may not develop until the child has lived through two or three ragweed seasons.

7. Can children outgrow allergies?

Children do tend to get better as they get older. However, some keep their allergies most of their lives. although usually in a milder form. Unfortunately doctors can't tell whether or not your child will ''grow out'' of his or her allergies or when this might happen.

8. Can allergies be caused by emotional problems?

It was once felt that emotional problems played a significant role in allergies. Today we believe that while physical manifestations of emotions, such as laughing or crying may cause rapid breathing which may in turn cause wheezing (especially in a child whose asthma is not under control), the emotions themselves do *not* cause allergic problems. Certainly children who have problems with allergies may be emotionally distressed and need support to live as normal a life as possible. They should not be made to feel guilty because some things have to be adjusted in the home setting, and the family must be careful not to make them feel that they are to blame for their problem.

9. What is Twentieth Century Disease?

This term has been coined by a new type of physician, the clinical ecologist. According to clinical ecologists, each person exists in dynamic equilibrium with his or her environment. Over a long period of time an imbalance can occur. This imbalance may be triggered by infections, major stress or exposure to toxic chemicals, either in large doses or in lower doses over longer periods of time.

Clinical ecologists maintain that a wide variety of problems result from such an imbalance, for example behaviour disorders, migraine headaches, depression, chronic fatigue, arthritis, hypertension, learning disabilities, schizophrenia, stomach upsets, chest problems and urinary complaints. In fact there are very few problems which have not been linked to such imbalances. In short, the clinical ecologist has widened the definition of allergy.

Traditional allergy organizations such as the American Academy of Allergy are concerned that some of the testing done to prove these associations and the treatments recommended are not scientifically valid. Allergists agree that many things in the environment may affect us adversely, but do not agree that the mechanisms involved in all of them are necessarily allergic. In order to prove the cause of such problems, carefully controlled scientific studies rather than chance observations are required, a principle which the Hospital for Sick Children endorses. By wrongly identifying the cause of such illnesses as schizophrenia, arthritis, cancer and so on, we may do harm with our treatments and keep people from seeking more appropriate help.

10. How are allergies treated?

Allergies are treated in three ways:

- **Drugs:** There are numerous medications available to both prevent, and provide relief from, allergic problems. Some children require occasional use of these drugs and others require much more long-term drug therapy.
- **Allergy injections** help some people who are allergic to specific unavoidable things in their environment such as pollen from trees, grass or weeds.
- **Changing the environment** is a major form of treatment. It is very important to reduce your child's exposure to the allergens that cause problems and also to the things that may irritate him or her, such as cigarette smoke and chemicals. Controlling your child's environment may reduce the need for medication or allergy injections.

Details about each of these treatment methods will be discussed in subsequent chapters.

2

Does your child have allergies?

The following problems may indicate that your child has allergies. Since each may be caused by another disease, you should consult with your doctor to make sure allergies are responsible before taking any further steps.

Frequent colds

Most children will have six to eight colds in their first two years of life and three to four per year in their third and fourth years. (Children who attend nurseries or daycare centres often have more colds because they are exposed to other children's colds.) If, however, your child's colds last longer than several weeks and/or your child always seems to have a cold, allergies may be the reason.

Frequent ear infections

Many children have this problem. Although allergies are not always the cause, it is a possibility worth investigating.

Sniffing, snoring and mouth breathing

Parents often think that sniffing, snoring and mouth breathing are simply bad habits caused by not blowing one's nose properly. This isn't always the case. If these signs persist for weeks or months, they may indicate that the lining of the nose is swollen because of allergies.

Watery liquid from the nose and/or sneezing

A cold could be the cause of this watery liquid, but if it persists, it may be a sign of allergies.

Itching or rubbing of the nose

Chances are children who are constantly rubbing their noses are not doing so out of habit. They may be trying to unblock a congested nasal passage to allow freer breathing. Rubbing the nose is such a familiar hallmark of an allergy sufferer that it has been nicknamed "the allergic salute." If it is done repeatedly, it may even produce a crease across the nose which is called "the allergic crease."

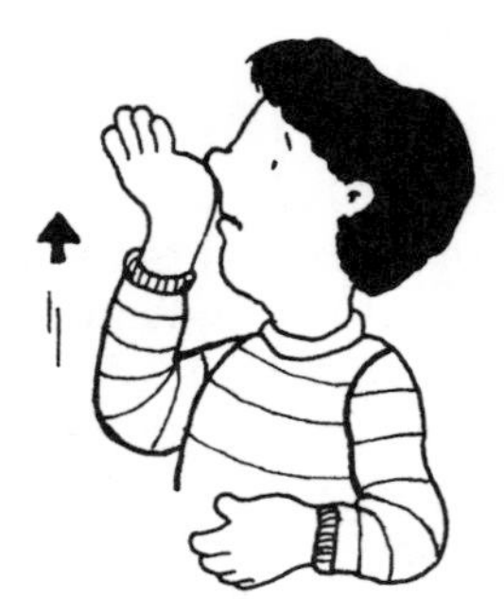

The allergic salute

Repeated nose bleeds

The blood vessels at the tip of the nose are quite near the surface of the skin. Allergies may cause the lining of the nose to swell, and this in turn can disturb these surface blood vessels, breaking them and causing nose bleeds.

Frequent throat clearing and/or coughing

Repeated throat clearing, especially when the child wakes up in the morning, may be caused by allergies. Allergies cause the nose to swell and fill with mucus. Then either the mucus drips down through the back of the nasal passage into the throat, causing the child to clear his or her throat, or the throat becomes dry because the mucus-clogged nose cannot moisten the air that is being breathed in. When the latter happens, the back of the throat becomes irritated, causing coughing.

Headaches

Frequent headaches, especially in the front part of the head near the nose, may indicate allergies. Headaches occur because of pressure caused by the swelling in the nose. Or the sinuses may be affected. These are hollow cavities in the skull just above the nose and connected to it. Congestion in the nose can spread to the sinuses.

Coughing

Coughing may be a mild form of asthma. If coughing has persisted for months, is worse at night or is aggravated by smoke, cold air or exercise, asthma, an allergic reaction of the lungs, may be the cause.

Wheezing, rapid breathing, chest congestion

All of these may be caused by lung diseases such as bronchitis, bronchiolitis or pneumonia. However, if these signs recur more than three or four times, asthma should be considered.

Breathing difficulties or coughing with exercise or laughing

If your child repeatedly develops coughing and/or difficulty breathing after any sort of exertion, including laughing or crying, this may indicate an underlying asthmatic problem.

Eye redness, watery discharge and/or swelling

Eye problems can be caused by infections, but if they occur repeatedly, especially during the allergy season (spring, summer and fall), allergies may be the cause.

Dark circles under the eyes

In many cases, fatigue or family genes may cause dark circles. But in a large number of people, these circles, or "allergic shiners" as they are called, are the result of allergies. The colour comes when blood moves more slowly than normal through the veins under the eyes.

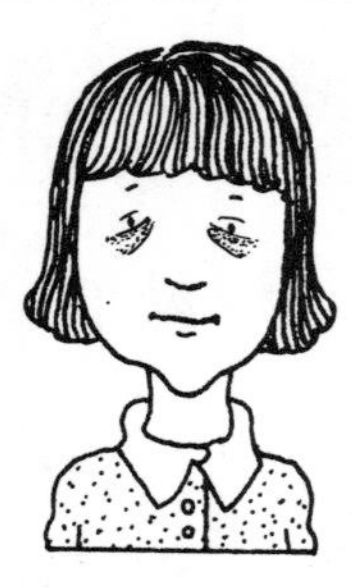

Allergic shiners

This happens when a blockage in the nose causes a back-up in the veins.

Facial changes

Children who have long-standing nose obstruction may develop a high arched palate or narrow chin and an overbite.

Skin rashes

There are two main types of rashes caused by allergies. **Eczema** may cause reddened itchy areas that ooze, scratch marks, bleeding, infected looking skin or thickened areas with fissures, scaling and darker than normal colouring. In infants these rashes often appear on the cheeks, scalp, neck, back of the arms, front of the legs and trunk. In the older child, common problem areas are the knee and elbow creases, neck, wrists and ankles.

Hives, or urticaria, are reddened swellings of the skin which are itchy and turn white when pressure is applied. Individual patches vary from dime-sized or smaller to much larger when several patches join together. There may also be swelling on the face, eyes, lips, hands, feet or genitalia.

Vomiting and diarrhea

Because there are numerous possible causes for vomiting and diarrhea, allergies should only be considered if there is a definite and consistent connection to certain foods.

Adenoid and tonsil problems

Repeated swellings inside the nose, caused by allergies, may allow infections to develop more easily. These infections may spread to the adenoids, which are located at the back of the nose, and cause them to swell, blocking the nasal passage. Surgically removing the adenoids may alleviate the obstruction caused by the allergic nose problem, but it will not cure the allergy.

The tonsils are located at the back of the throat and their purpose is to protect against infection. Unfortunately they may be so overrun by infections that they are no longer useful and become swollen. These repeated infections are not due to allergies and hence their removal does not help the allergic problem. Today we know that adenoids and tonsils help to fight infection, and we only remove them as a last resort.

3

Investigating your child's allergy problem

Children who develop sensitivity to certain allergens such as dust or animals also tend to be sensitive to other factors such as cold weather or pollution. They become *hypersensitive*. Because of this, it is sometimes difficult to isolate the cause of the allergy. Here's what you can do to help.

Provide a complete history

To help your doctor's investigation, write down observations and questions about your child's condition before the visit. The following are just a few of the questions your doctor might ask:

- When did your child's problem first start?
- How often does it bother the child?
- How long does each attack last or is the child always ill?
- What time of the day is the worst?
- What time of year is the worst?
- Where is the problem worse: at home, outside, other buildings, countryside, vacation areas and so on?
- What makes the child's problem worse?
- Do your child's symptoms change with physical changes such as cold, heat, dampness or with exercise or exposure to cigarette smoke?
- What treatments, including drugs, have been tried?
- What treatments or drugs have worked best?
- What allergic problems are present in other members of the family?
- Does your child have other medical problems?
- What other illnesses has your child had in the past?

Keep a diary

Many people think that allergic reactions occur immediately on contact with an allergen, for example, sneezing as soon as a child starts to play with a cat. But reactions can occur several hours after the contact.

For this reason keeping a diary is most helpful. If a child becomes ill with an allergic reaction in the evening, one should not only record what he or she is in contact with at the time, but what he or she was doing a few hours earlier, such as playing out in the cold, playing with a cat or whatever. Even noting if the weather changed rapidly or if it was damp outside is important. Complete recordings will enable you to note similar patterns in your child's illness, and your doctor will then be in a better position to advise you.

Testing for allergies

With the aid of information you provide, your doctor will try to narrow the cause of the problem. Often he or she will order laboratory tests. These tests alone will not allow your doctor to pinpoint the cause — many other diseases can cause the test results to be abnormal — but they will serve as clues to unravelling your child's problem.

Skin tests

This is one of the major tests used by allergists. Special drops containing possible allergens such as ragweed, dust, mould and so on are placed on your child's back or, in the older child, on the forearm. The skin is then pricked with a needle allowing the allergen to enter the skin. This is referred to as the **prick test**. In a **scratch test** a linear scratch is made in the skin very superficially and a drop of possible allergen is placed on the scratch. In both tests an area of redness with some swelling in the middle will develop if the child is allergic to the substance. This reaction takes place about 15 to 30 minutes after the testing and is usually quite harmless. If a severe reaction develops, the allergen can be wiped off the skin.

Another form of skin test consists of injecting the allergen into the outer skin of the upper half of the arm. This is called an **intradermal test**. It is used when the prick test does not show a reaction. Intradermal tests are often overly sensitive and may identify factors that your child is not actually allergic to. For this reason it is only used in select cases and requires careful interpretation by your doctor.

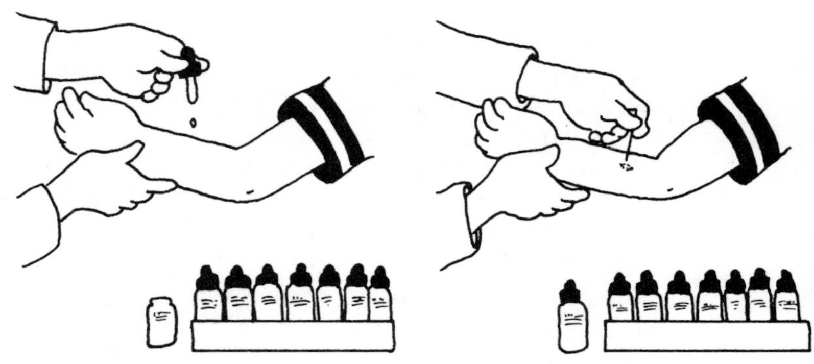

The prick test: an allergen drop is placed on the arm, then the arm is pricked with a needle.

Sometimes skin tests cannot be used. For example, if the child reacts to everything that is tested, his or her skin may be too sensitive for a skin test. Or if the child's skin is covered with eczema, a skin test may not be advisable. In these cases the Rast test (described below) might be used instead.

Skin tests have their limitations, but they have stood the test of time and serve as a reliable indicator of allergies. Because children grow and change and are constantly exposed to new things in the environment, their allergies can change as they get older. For this reason skin testing may be repeated every few years if the child is still having problems.

Skin tests are usually done for children age three or older, although they can be done at a younger age if the child is having severe problems. This is because it may take two or three allergy seasons before the child develops a reaction to a particular allergen. Only then will it show up on skin tests.

Blood tests

Eosinophil count: The eosinophil is a cell in the body that helps defend against allergic reactions. It is brought to the site of the allergic reaction by the blood. During an allergic response the number of eosinophils in the blood may increase. An elevated eosinophil count may therefore indicate an allergy.

Total IgE count: When a foreign substance, or allergen, enters the body, antibodies are produced. Allergic antibodies are called IgE. If IgE levels in the blood are elevated, the patient may have an allergic problem.

Rast test: This test measures not the total IgE, but the amount of specific IgE that is being built up in the body against a specific antigen such as ragweed or grass pollen. A Rast test provides the same information as a skin test. Because it is no more (or less) accurate than the skin test, and because it is expensive, it is not routinely done. It can be used in patients where there are difficulties in performing the skin test.

Histamine release test: The mast cells lining the nose, lungs and skin release certain chemicals when the allergic reaction occurs. One of the chemicals released is histamine. The amount of histamine released indicates how sensitive the child is to a substance. This test, however, is time-consuming, expensive and only done in research laboratories.

Challenge testing

In selected cases the allergen may be given to the child directly into the nose or eye or breathed directly into the lungs. The subsequent reaction is then measured on special machines. Because it is time-consuming and costly and can only be done by trained personnel, challenge testing is only used for research purposes.

Other tests

There are many different tests that your allergist may perform in order to rule out other disorders that can mimic the allergic condition. These will be discussed in subsequent sections.

Tests of questionable value

Some of the allergy tests discussed above were developed before good scientific tests could prove their validity. Over the years, however, they have been validated by proper scientific evaluations.

Other types of allergy tests have *not* measured up to the same standards. Since you would not accept lower standards for the drugs that your child takes, you should not accept lower standards for the tests used to diagnose his or her illness. The following tests have not yet met acceptable scientific testing requirements.

Cytotoxicity testing (Leukocytic food allergy test): This test claims to identify specific food allergies by observing the changes in, and apparent size and shape of, white blood cells when a food is added to a blood sample. The American Academy of Allergy has found cytotoxicity testing to be unreliable and without scientific basis. It is also time-consuming and costly. The U.S. Food and Drug Administration has banned it.

Sublingual food drops: In these tests the patient is given the suspect food as drops under the tongue. If symptoms develop, the patient is then given weaker doses of the food in order to ''neutralize'' or stop the reaction. If a specific food is discovered to be the problem, the treatment is either avoidance of the food or administration of food drops under the tongue before or after eating the suspect food. This technique has been investigated and found to be of questionable value by the American Academy of Allergy, the American College of Allergists and the Asthma and Allergy Foundation of America.

4

Allergic rhinitis and hay fever

Allergic rhinitis, or catarrh as it is called in Britain, could be described as one cold after another. It involves a recurring runny, stuffy, itchy nose and frequent sneezing. Often the eyes are itchy, red and watery. These symptoms are the result of an allergic reaction in the mucous membrane or lining of the nose and/or eye.

About 1.6-million Canadians have allergic rhinitis and 25 per cent of them are children. Equal numbers of boys and girls are affected. Heredity may play a role as it does with other allergic diseases, but it isn't possible to predict which child in a family is likely to develop this condition and at what age.

There are two main types of allergic rhinitis. **Perennial allergic rhinitis** occurs all year round. It is usually caused by house dust, animal danders, moulds and aggravated by irritants such as pollution and tobacco smoke. **Seasonal allergic rhinitis**, also called **hay fever**, occurs in the spring and early summer or in the fall. It may affect the eyes even more than the nose. In the spring and early summer it is usually caused by pollen from trees and grass and spring mould spores. In the autumn it is caused by pollen from ragweed and fall mould spores.

What causes allergic rhinitis?

The lining of the nose is affected by colds and allergic factors just as the lungs are. In young children, dust, animals and possibly foods tend to cause inflammation in the nose. (Foods do not play as big a role as many people have felt in the past and the importance of foods tends to decline as the child ages.) However, after several allergy seasons, the child's nose may become sensitized to new allergens such as tree, grass or ragweed pollens.

At any age, irritants such as dry air, tobacco, pollution, rapid weather changes, humidity, cosmetics, perfumes might trigger reactions in the nose. These irritants act on an already hypersensitive nose which has become "twitchy" because of the inflammatory changes due to the allergic reactions.

When to suspect allergic rhinitis

Your child may have any or all of the following:

- watery discharge from the nose all the time, occasionally or at certain seasons of the year
- stuffy nose all the time or at specific seasons
- reddened, pebbly lining in the lower eyelids
- frequent throat-clearing
- breathing through the mouth
- snoring
- rabbit-like movements of the nose
- a horizontal crease across the nose about 1 centimetre (½ inch) from the tip as a result of rubbing the nose upward with the palm of the hand
- bouts of sneezing, especially in the morning
- repeated nosebleeds
- headaches because of pressure from inside the nose or actual spread of infection into the sinuses
- frequent earaches or ear infections, occasional hearing loss with buzzing and popping sounds, a feeling of fullness in the ears
- dizziness or nausea related to ear problems
- chronic cold without much fever but with a scratchy throat
- nasal tone to the voice because of mouth breathing and blocked nasal passages
- dark circles under the eyes as a result of pressure from the blocked nasal passages on the small blood vessels. (This is not related to lack of sleep as some parents suspect.)

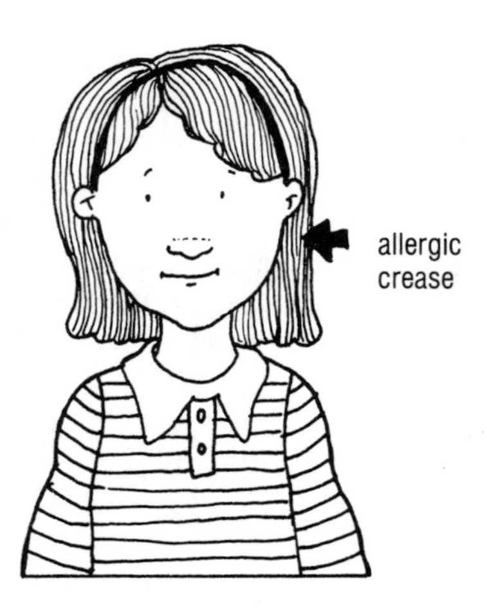

Determining the causes of allergic rhinitis

History

The doctor will need a complete history of the child's condition, including information on how often the child has this problem, whether there is any seasonal variation to it, what effect the environment has on it, and what the family history is. You can come prepared by answering these and other questions on page 16 and by keeping a diary (see page 16).

Physical examination

After taking a thorough history, the doctor will do a physical examination. In particular he or she will be concerned about the appearance of the nose, eyes, ears and throat. The doctor will also be looking for evidence of other allergic problems such as skin rashes, asthma and so on.

Tests

Allergy skin tests may be done to confirm if there are any specific allergies. These tests are described on page 17. X-rays may also be taken to determine if the sinuses are involved and/or if the adenoids are swollen. (X-rays are not required in every patient.) The sinuses are cavities in the skull that are connected to the nasal passages. Congestion in the nose may extend into the sinuses and adenoids causing complications requiring extra medication or removal of the adenoids for some children.

How allergic rhinitis is treated

Reduce your child's contact with the irritant

There are many things you can do to change your child's environment to reduce contact with irritants. Details are explained in *Coping with the environment*, chapter 10.

Drugs

Antihistamines are used to alleviate the symptoms of allergic rhinitis. They may also be used for other allergic problems such as hives or eczema. They are available in pill, time-release capsules or liquid form and can also be given by injection or as creams.

Antihistamines work by blocking the action of a chemical called histamine, which is released by allergically sensitized tissues. It is best to give antihistamines before the allergic reaction or as early as possible. Giving such medicines before an allergic reaction is obviously difficult. However, if the child is having frequent problems, these drugs can be given daily for a few weeks as necessary or even during an entire allergy season.

The major side effect of antihistamines is sedation. Some antihistamines are more likely to cause this than others. Sometimes this drowsiness may lessen after a few days. When it persists, you should inform your doctor. He or she may recommend a change in the dosage or drug prescribed.

A partial list of other side effects includes excitability, irritability, nightmares, dry mouth, fever, bruising or unusual bleeding, tiredness or weakness. These can add to the effects of alcohol, sleeping pills or tranquillizers. Hence caution is advised if these other drugs are taken.

There are numerous antihistamines available. Some are used only in certain situations. For example, Periactin is often prescribed for hives caused by exposure to cold. In most cases, however, allergic problems will respond to many different antihistamines and so the doctor will try to give preparations with the least side effects. It may be necessary to try two or three different antihistamines before success is achieved.

Some commonly available antihistamines are Atarax,

Benadryl, Chlortripolon, Periactin, Phenergan, Tavist, Seldane and Hismanal.

The two newest preparations — Seldane and Hismanal — are better for children because they cause less drowsiness than other preparations and do not have to be given as frequently. Seldane is available in liquid or tablet form and is administered twice a day. It may cause slight headaches or stomach upsets. Hismanal is available in drops or tablet form and is given once per day on an empty stomach. If taken over a prolonged period, it may cause an increased appetite and weight gain.

Decongestants help to shrink the swollen membranes in the nose which makes it easier for the child to breathe. They may be used to reduce the swellings caused by colds or allergies.

Side effects include drowsiness or irritability, and decongestants may interact with other medications such as drugs for thyroid disease, diabetes, high blood pressure, depression or heart disease.

Decongestants come in pure preparations such as Sudafed or in combination with antihistamines in such drugs as Dimetapp, Triaminic and Novahistine, to name a few. As with the antihistamines, changes may be needed to find the right drug for the child.

Today with the new, purer and safer antihistamine preparations available, some of the above combination drugs may not be used as often, especially if the reaction in the nose is purely an allergic one.

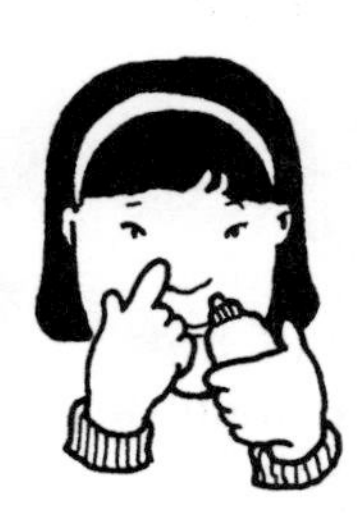

Block one nostril while inhaling nasal spray

Nasal sprays: Some decongestant sprays, such as Otrivin and Neo-synephrine, are used to relieve short-duration nasal congestion lasting for less than one week. Prolonged use of these preparations may result in worsening of the nasal congestion.

New nasal sprays do not cause this problem and are felt to be quite safe. Among these are Beconase, Vancenase and Rhinalar. These are steroid preparations which are used in a preventive manner. For example, they may be used for weeks or months at a time during an allergy season. Many people associate steroids with the side effects of oral steroids, but such side effects are very unlikely with inhaled steroids as long as the dosage prescribed is adhered to and the child is taking the spray correctly.

Another spray called Rynacrom is actually the same

drug as Intal, which is used for the asthmatic patient. It too is a preventative drug and is used in a similar fashion to the steroid inhalers. The dose is usually one to two inhalations, two to four times a day.

There may be stinging, burning, nasal irritation, nosebleed, sneezing, throat irritation or sore throat with nasal sprays. And Rynacrom may produce some rashes on the skin. It may also produce sneezing, coughing, headache and, occasionally, pneumonia. These side effects are very rare and can be controlled either by decreasing the dose or stopping the medication. Nasal sprays can be used along with antihistamines or decongestants.

Eye drops: The eye problems that sometimes occur with allergic rhinitis may not always respond to the above medications. Drops can be used as well.

Eye drops containing decongestants alone or in combination with antihistamines are available for mild to moderate eye problems. Eye irritation is one side effect.

Steroid eye drops are used more rarely, for severe eye problems. If steroid eye drops are needed for more than a few days, their use should be supervised by an eye specialist.

A newer, safer preparation is Opticrom (which is sodium cromoglycate). It is the same preparation that is used in Intal for asthma and Rynacrom for allergic rhinitis. It seems to be quite effective for allergic eye problems. Usually one drop, two to four times a day, is required to help with the eye problem.

Immunotherapy

As the name implies, immunotherapy is a type of immunization. The allergist orders an extract that includes the major allergens as determined by allergy skin testing. Foods and other substances your child can avoid, such as animals, are not included. Small amounts of this extract are injected at regular intervals, and the dose is increased as tolerated. In response to these injections the child's body forms antibodies to the allergens. Eventually the antibody level is sufficient to control the symptoms caused by exposure to the allergens.

The injections are given weekly for at least a year. As

the child improves, the interval between injections is gradually increased to a month.

Allergy injections of this kind should not cause more than brief swelling, redness or soreness where the needle went in. If any other problem occurs, the allergist must be told so that the extract can be diluted.

When the child has been on monthly injections for a year or so without a relapse, he or she is ready to try stopping the injections. Many children are successfully weaned off the injections, but others require them for years. If a relapse occurs either during or after treatment, the allergist will reassess the child's situation and repeat skin tests. This may be necessary because new allergens affect children as they mature and their environments change.

New extracts have been developed that allow the allergy treatment to be given before the allergy season, and fewer injections are required. This method is used more in older children and adults and is not applicable to everyone. Medical advice is necessary to determine which type of immunotherapy is best for your child.

5

Asthma

Asthma is an allergy-related disease that involves intermittent bouts of coughing, wheezing and breathing difficulty because of a narrowing of the breathing tubes leading into the lungs. This narrowing is caused when the lining of the tubes becomes inflamed and swells, the muscles in the walls of the tubes go into spasm and the tubes fill up with phlegm or mucus. A whistling or wheezing sound may be produced when air moves through these narrowed tubes.

Asthmatic children are born with sensitive breathing tubes (bronchi) which, at some point in the child's life, begin to react to things in the environment such as allergens or viruses. Once this happens, the child begins to cough or wheeze frequently.

We know that this tendency is inherited. If you or your spouse have asthma, your child is more likely to develop asthma too. But exactly why it affects some children and not others in the same family is not understood.

When should you suspect asthma?

If your child wheezes as he or she breathes, asthma may be the cause. But there are other symptoms to watch for as well. Frequent or extended periods of coughing and chest rattling, or "chestiness," may be

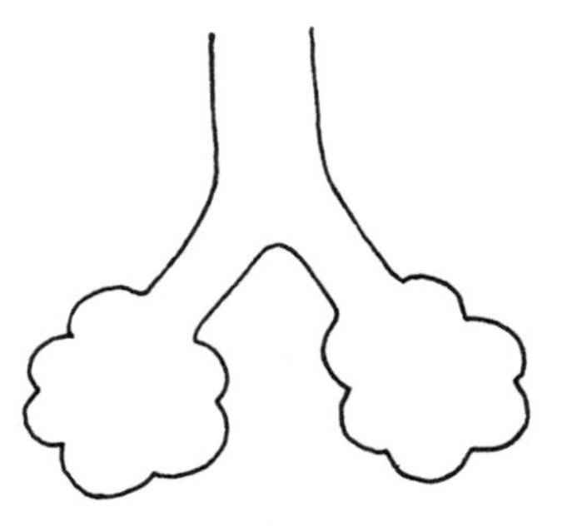

Normal breathing tubes (bronchi)

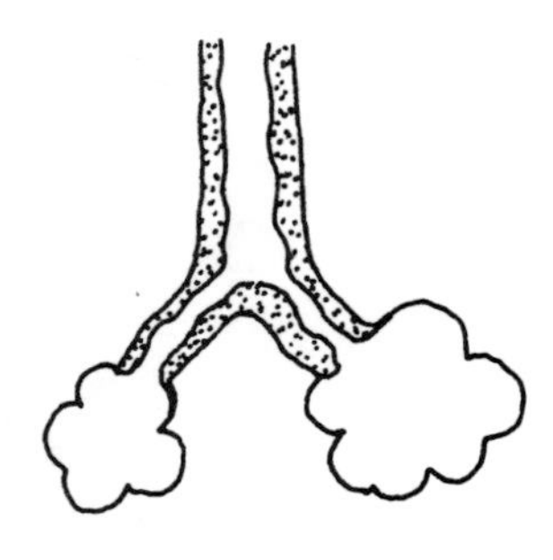

Narrowed bronchi in an asthmatic

asthma signals. And children who are repeatedly diagnosed as having bronchitis or pneumonia and show no improvement when treated with antibiotics may also have asthma. Finally, children who have other allergic problems such as eczema or hay fever and then develop prolonged or frequent bouts of coughing or wheezing should be suspected of having asthma.

Many parents first learn of their child's asthma after an asthma attack that requires medical attention. During an asthma attack the child's chest may move in and out rapidly, there may be a sucking in and out of the muscles between the ribs and also above the collar bones. The muscles running between the collar bones and the base of the jaw may be quite prominent. The child's lips may appear blue, and there may be coughing, whistling sounds or wheezing as the child tries to breathe out. Asthma is not the only illness that can produce these reactions, but it is one of the most likely causes.

Asthma is a common childhood disease, compared with other diseases. For example, diabetes affects 1 to 2 per cent of children, whereas asthma affects 5 to 10 per cent.

How asthma is diagnosed

When you take your child to the doctor the first step will be to compile a complete history of the symptoms to date. You can greatly assist your doctor by observing your child's condition and keeping detailed records of it. For more information on how to do this, see page 16.

Many tests may be ordered by your doctor to determine if your child has allergies, since allergies and asthma are related in some children. Many of these tests are described on pages 17 to 19. Some of the following tests may also be done if the child is wheezing.

Chest x-ray

X-rays are taken primarily to rule out other rare causes of wheezing or complications of asthma such as chest infection. Repeated chest x-rays are not needed.

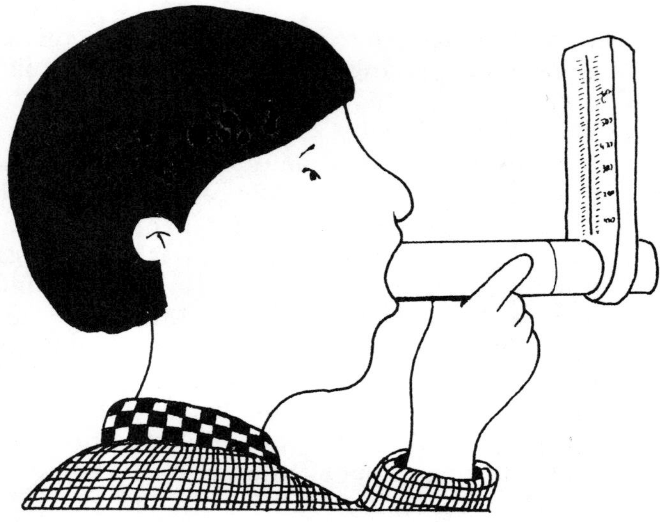

The peak flow meter

Lung function tests

A child over age seven may be tested for asthma by having him or her breathe into a machine that monitors lung functions. In some tests, breathing patterns are used to diagnose asthma. In others, the speed at which air is forced out of the lungs is measured. (In an asthmatic, air does not flow out as fast as in the normal child.)

These tests allow doctors to measure the severity of the disease. A repeat test after treatment can measure the effectiveness of the treatment. One lung testing instrument is the peak flow meter. It can also be used at home, thus enabling the parent to chart changes in the child's asthma both with and without treatment.

Lung function tests should be performed when the diagnosis of asthma is not certain or when there is a problem in management.

Upper GI series

In this test, a milk-like fluid called barium is given to your child to drink and x-rays are taken as the fluid moves through the esophagus. Abnormal blood vessels or other structures pressing against your child's windpipe and producing wheezing can be seen.

Some children are unable to pass all their food into the stomach. Some of it comes back into the throat and is inhaled into the lungs, producing wheezing. This can be identified by an upper GI series as well. These are rare causes of wheezing and hence this test is not routinely done.

Sweat chloride tests

Other diseases, such as cystic fibrosis, can involve wheezing. However, children with cystic fibrosis usually also have diarrhea and have difficulty gaining weight. By measuring the amount of sweat released on the back a doctor can rule out this more serious condition.

Blood antibody (immunoglobulin) levels

Certain proteins called immunoglobulins are essential for protecting us against infection. Measuring their levels will help the doctor determine whether they are high enough to fight infection. One such protein, IgE, is actually elevated if the person is highly allergic. Children who are wheezing and have high IgE levels are more likely to have asthma.

Patterns of asthmatic attacks

Asthma varies greatly in severity. Some asthmatics have very sensitive airways and seem to wheeze after the slightest stimulus. They have frequent attacks, as often as every few weeks or even daily. Others wheeze only after very strong stimulation. Even two children with asthma in the same family may not have it to the same degree. Some children's attacks may last for days or weeks at a time, while others only for a few hours.

Most asthma is mild and easily managed. Twenty to 30 per cent of children "outgrow" their asthma, and another 30 per cent improve as they get older. The remaining 30 per cent — usually those who have severe asthma in early childhood — continue to have problems with asthma as adults. Today, fortunately, there are medications that can greatly assist these people in coping with their disease.

Deaths from asthma are very rare indeed, and severe disability from asthma is no longer common. Most children should be able to do everything all other children do: grow, thrive, play sports, attend school, visit the country and so on.

What makes asthma worse?

Two major factors, allergies and viral infections, cause asthma by increasing inflammation of the lungs and thereby increasing the airway sensitivity. Other factors do not actually *cause* asthma but may bring out asthma that is not under control. In other words, other factors may irritate already twitchy or hypersensitive airways. These factors include: cold air, rapid changes in temperature, humidity, cigarette smoke, exercise, indoor or outdoor pollution, time of day (such as night time, early morning), drugs such as Aspirin, foods, food additives such as sulfites and even emotions in some cases.

Viral infections such as colds

Viruses are the most common causes of infections such as colds in young children. They also are the most common cause of asthmatic attacks, especially in children under age five. Viruses are very widespread in the community all year round and are difficult to avoid. Antibiotics are ineffective against them. (Bacteria on the other hand are larger bugs. They cause such conditions as strep throat, which *do* respond to antibiotics.)

Children normally have six to eight colds a year in the first two years of life. They may have more frequent colds if they attend day care centres or have frequent contact with other children. If the child is an ashmatic, colds may precipitate wheezing attacks. This is why your doctor may advise you to start anti-asthmatic medications at the beginning of a cold rather than waiting for any wheezing to start. By doing so it is hoped that most attacks can be prevented.

Allergies

Allergens are a significant cause of asthma, especially in younger children. For example, at least one allergen is involved in causing attacks in 98 per cent of children who acquire asthma by age ten and in 92 per cent of people who acquire asthma between 11 and 20 years of age. As people get older allergens are less likely to be involved. Only 29 per cent of people who first develop asthma after age 60 have attacks that are caused by allergens.

Allergens abound in the environment, but certain ones are more likely to cause problems at certain ages simply because of the degree of exposure. The infant or young child is likely to be affected by foods such as milk, eggs, fish, nuts or peanuts or by household dust and animal dander. In older children who have experienced several allergy seasons, pollen grains from trees, grasses and weeds as well as moulds are more likely to be the cause.

Exercise

Exercise often exacerbates asthma in children. The attack usually starts five to six minutes after the exercise begins and is more severe after the exercise is over. Attacks may last up to 20 minutes. Occasionally they go on for several hours. The child may not always wheeze during an attack; coughing and/or chest tightness may be the predominant feature. This may result from breathing cold dry air during the exercise. Running in cold weather is a common cause of exercise-induced asthma. Swimming is less frequently a cause of this problem.

Exercise causes a significant problem for some asthmatic children. They may be unable to participate in competitive sports or may need medication in order to take part. These medications (discussed in the treatment section) can be given one-half hour before exercising.

Asthmatic children should not avoid exercise. They should take part in school physical education programs as much as possible. This will both help them "fit in" and strengthen their growing heart and lungs. However, it may be necessary to discuss your child's condition with his or her physical education teacher. This will allow you to ensure that pre-medication is correctly undertaken and that the child is neither pushed into over-exertion or excused from exercise.

Weather and pollution

Cold air is a strong stimulus for coughing and/or wheezing in asthmatics. This may be because cold air dries the lining of the breathing tubes. Rapid changes in temperature and/or humidity and increased humidity indoors or out can also irritate the asthmatic's lungs, as can pollutants such as cigarette smoke. Outdoor pollutants such as carbon monoxide and sulfur dioxide may contribute to asthma too. They do not directly cause wheezing but are triggers that act on sensitive lungs.

Time of day

Coughing and/or wheezing is sometimes worse at night or in the morning. This is a problem for asthmatics because mucus builds up in the night so that sleep is eventually disturbed.

Occasionally the environment in the bedroom may exacerbate asthma. See page 75 for some suggestions on how to improve the bedroom environment.

Drugs

A few drugs may cause problems for asthmatics. For example, some drugs used to fight arthritis, including Aspirin, may affect some asthmatics. In some cases severe attacks can be produced by even one tablet. Why this happens is not known; possibly Aspirin blocks certain chemicals that help fight off asthmatic attacks. Because of this, asthmatics should use other drugs for fever and/or pain control, such as acetaminophen products (Tylenol or Tempra). Those who react to Aspirin may also have problems with yellow dye #5, or tartrazine, which is a colouring additive found in many foods. There does not appear to be as high an incidence of reaction to this dye in children as in adults but nevertheless it should not be ignored. (See page 57 for more information on food additives and allergies.)

Food and food additives

Foods such as milk may occasionally bring on bouts of wheezing. If wheezing occurs directly after ingesting a food, this information should be passed on to the doctor. He or she may recommend that the food be eliminated from the diet. However, no food should be removed from a diet just because it is suspect. Only your doctor should make that decision. Careless elimination of foods may impair a child's health. Foods, however, are not a very common cause of wheezing as compared to other factors.

Food additives, specifically preservatives such as sulfites, are found in high concentrations in restaurant foods such as salad bar salads, french fried potatoes and avocado dips. Ingestion of these preservatives by a small percentage of adult asthmatics (5-10 per cent) has produced severe wheezing within 30 minutes. The exact incidence in children is not known. For more information on sulfites and asthma, see the section on food allergies, page 59.

Emotions and asthma

Emotions are not as big a factor in provoking asthma attacks as was once felt. Today we no longer feel that statements such as "it is all in the child's head" are correct. Emotional upsets such as worrying about exams do not really provoke asthma attacks. However, emotional responses such as crying or laughing will cause the chest wall to move in and out and this physical motion may initiate an attack. Another way in which emotions may affect the asthmatic is if the child becomes upset and intentionally does not take the prescribed medication. Coping with the emotions is explored more thoroughly in chapter 11.

Asthma treatment

There are several ways in which asthma is treated. The two main ways are drug therapy and changing the child's immediate environment. Immunotherapy, diet and breathing exercises may also be used. Let's look at each in more detail.

Drug therapy

Today drugs are the major form of treatment for the asthmatic. There are many to choose from and they do not have long-term harmful side effects, nor are they addictive. They do, however, have side effects which may require alteration in dosage or a change in drugs.

Some children may need only one or several drugs intermittently; others may need one or several drugs on a daily basis for months or even a few years.

There are two main groups of asthma drugs: **bronchodilators** which treat the wheezing, and **preventative drugs** which are given daily to reduce the number of attacks. Neither group is 100 per cent effective alone and hence will be used in different combinations by your doctor.

Bronchodilators

These drugs help to open up the breathing (bronchial) tubes by relaxing the muscles that are in spasm in the walls of the tubes. There are three types: the beta-adrenergic drugs, theophylline compounds and anti-cholinergic medications. All achieve the same end result of muscle relaxation but by different mechanisms.

Beta-adrenergic drugs include the following: salbutamol (Ventolin), metaproterenol (Alupent), fenoterol (Berotec) and terbutaline (Bricanyl). These drugs can be

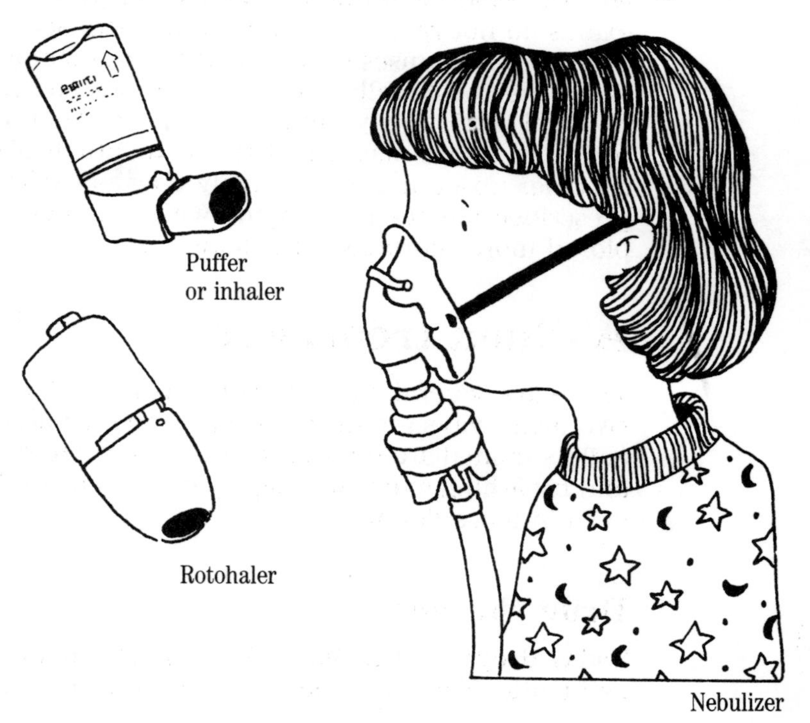

given by mouth (as tablets or liquid) or by inhalation using a metered dose inhaler (puffer) or small air compressor (nebulizer). Inhaling is preferable because the drugs work more rapidly, usually within five minutes. The effect of inhaled drugs usually lasts for three to four hours and they are associated with fewer side effects because the dose is lower.

Beta-adrenergic drugs can be used to stop an asthma attack. They can be given one to four times a day in a 24 hour period for an isolated attack or daily if the child has continuous wheezing. Beta-adrenergic drugs taken fifteen to thirty minutes before exercising or visiting areas where irritants or allergens abound may also serve as a means of protection. The maximum number of times they can be used is four times in 24 hours. If needed more often, medical help should be obtained.

These drugs may produce fine muscle tremors which last up to an hour or rapid heart beat. Both of these side effects can be controlled by lowering the dose. None of the drugs has any serious long-term effects on the body generally or on the heart in particular, and none is addictive.

Theophylline drugs are best used when daily medications are required for control. There are rapid acting forms such as Choledyl, Quibron and Somophyllin which must be given every six hours and are available in tablet or liquid form. Longer-acting forms are now available for more effective control. These can be taken every 12 hours. For children who have difficulty swallowing large pills there are two alternatives: Theo-Dur is a tablet which can be split in half and Somophyllin-12 is a capsule, the beads of which can be put into soft foods such as apple sauce. In the near future we may have medications that need only be taken once a day.

The side effects of theophylline drugs include nausea, vomiting, headaches, nervousness, irritability and inability to sleep. These effects may occur when starting the drug or come on more slowly after several weeks. Blood levels can be measured and the dosage tailored to individuals. In children, lower doses are usually given first, then the dosage is gradually increased using blood levels as a guide. In some patients, though, side effects occur even with normal blood levels. Stopping the drug

Continued on page 40

Use of inhalers

The **metered dose inhaler** can best be used by children over age seven. It should be used as follows:

1. remove the cap
2. shake the inhaler
3. hold the inhaler upright
4. tilt the head back slightly
5. close the lips over the mouthpiece of the inhaler
6. begin to breathe in and then activate the inhaler. Inhale slowly and deeply
7. hold the breath for ten seconds
8. breathe out through the nose. Wait 30 seconds before taking another puff if needed.

How to use an inhaler

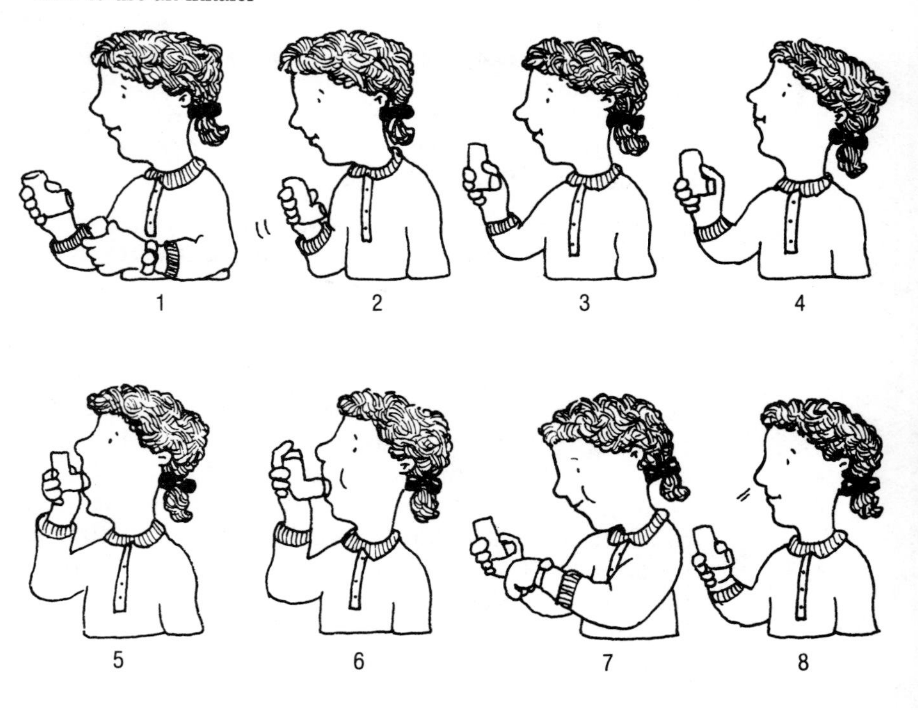

It is a good idea to have your doctor observe your child's use of the inhaler over several visits to ensure that it is being used correctly. Care of the inhaler is important and instructions are provided with the prescription.

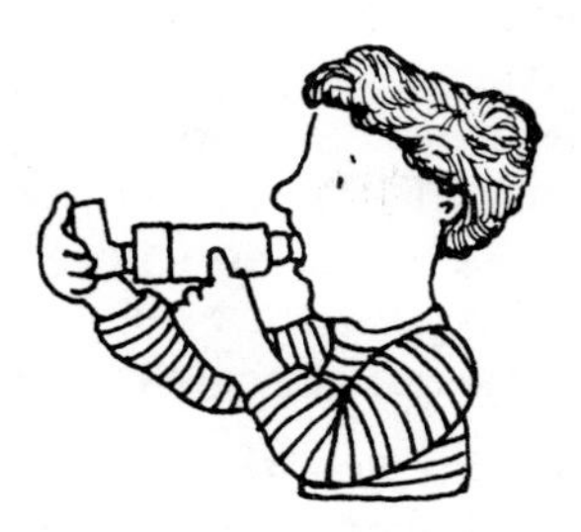

An aerochamber

For younger children (aged three to seven years) or those who have difficulty with the inhalers, there are longer tubes called **aerochambers** which can be attached to the inhalers. These hold the drug until the child is able to breathe it in.

There are also several other forms of inhalers called **rotohalers** which make it easier to inhale these drugs as well.

The **mask inhalation** technique via the **air compressor** is available for children under age four or for children who have severe attacks and cannot use the inhaler. Ventolin can be administered by placing a mask over the child's face. This can be done in hospital or at home. Special instructions as to use can be given by hospital personnel. Mask inhalation when given at home has helped to prevent many hospitalizations.

is the only way to see if it is indeed causing the problem. Blood tests should be taken every few months if the child is on these drugs for a prolonged period. Because of the frequent incidence of side effects with theophylline drugs, such as poor sleeping and poor appetite, the asthma clinic at the Hospital for Sick Children recommends inhaled beta-adrenergic drugs.

Anticholinergic drugs: Ipratropium bromide (Atrovent) is used mainly for adults and occasionally for children. It is given by inhalation only. Usually it is used for severe asthma which cannot be controlled by other medications. It can be used on a long-term basis or for a sudden attack. Its role in treating asthma in children is not well established. Side effects are minimal but include an unpleasant taste in the mouth.

Preventative drugs

Sodium Cromoglycate (Intal) prevents the release of chemicals that cause the breathing tubes to go into spasm. It is best used for children who have frequent attacks. In order to act as a preventative, it must be given two to four times a day, usually together with other medications such as Ventolin. It cannot be used to treat a sudden attack. However, children who use it daily need not stop using it when an attack occurs. In fact, it is often advantageous to give it four times a day along with the Ventolin at such a time. It may also be used to prevent exercise-induced wheezing if given 30 minutes prior to an activity.

This drug is available in special inhalers called spinhalers and halermatics, both of which use Intal capsules. There is also a metered dose inhaler available called Fivent. In addition, Intal is available as a solution

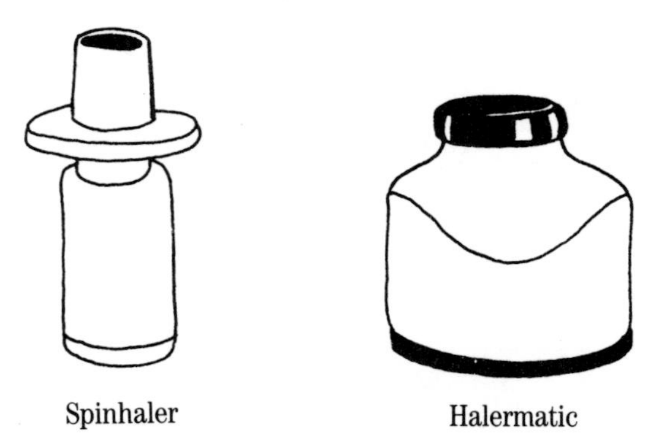

Spinhaler Halermatic

which can be given by air compressor. Side effects include minor coughing and wheezing after inhalation, but if Ventolin or other similar drug is given before the Intal, this problem can be overcome. Other side effects, which subside when the drug is discontinued, include hoarseness, nausea, vomiting, dizziness, hives and other skin rashes and pneumonia.

Steroids: The mechanism of how steroids work is not fully understood. We *do* know that they help to reduce inflammatory changes in the breathing tubes. This then allows the other medications to work more successfully. Steroids can be given orally (Prednisone tablets) for short periods (under two weeks) or intravenously (Solu-Cortef) for a few days, when the asthma is out of control. It is preferable not to use steroids on a daily, long-term basis for months at a time because they are associated with many unpleasant side effects related to growth and effects on the eyes, bones and other organs in the body. Occasionally steroids can be given in low doses every other morning in extremely severe patients, but this must be closely supervised by a physician.

Steroids can also be given by inhalation, either through an inhaler or a rotohaler in the form of beclomethasone (Beclovent or Vanceril). Beclomethasone acts locally on the breathing tubes. Very little is absorbed, and the side effects of oral steroids can be avoided. It is more effectively used, like Intal, on a preventative basis (that is, daily even when the patient is well and usually in combination with other medications mentioned previously). It will not help with a sudden attack on its own, but if it is already being used daily it need not be discontinued during the attack. Instead, it can be given along with Ventolin. Side effects may include a yeast infection in the mouth. This can be prevented by rinsing the mouth with water after taking an inhalation.

Environmental controls

Reducing your child's exposure to factors which aggravate his or her asthma is extremely important as this can help to reduce the amount of medication needed for control. How this can be achieved is discussed in *Coping with the environment*, chapter 10.

Immunotherapy

Immunotherapy (commonly called allergy shots) involves regular injections of an extract which contains substances (allergens) to which the child is allergic. The purpose of immunotherapy is to increase the child's resistance to the allergens by gradually increasing the strength of the injections. Eventually the child can tolerate enough of the allergen so that exposure to it in the environment no longer bothers him or her. If a child has very few allergies, immunotherapy can be very helpful. However, children with asthma often have a wide range of allergies, and there is little evidence that giving injections against multiple allergens improves their condition. As a result, immunotherapy is not appropriate for many children with asthma.

For children whose asthma is triggered by a few specific allergens which cannot be avoided, immunotherapy may be helpful. Skin testing is done to identify the allergens before the injections are started. The injections are given weekly for at least a year, and as improvement occurs they are reduced to once a month. Usually they are continued for three to five years. During this time the child must also take his or her regular asthma medications.

Diet

In some children foods may be involved in causing asthmatic attacks. However, foods are not as important a cause of asthma as was once believed. If a food such as strawberries causes wheezing shortly after it is eaten, it can be eliminated from your child's diet. However, these "elimination diets" must be carefully monitored by a nutritionist or nutritional deficiencies may result. For more information on elimination diets, see the section on food allergies on page 55.

Breathing exercises

Physiotherapists can instruct your child on breathing exercises to help control breathing in a mild attack so that he or she will not panic and make things worse.

Your child's future

Control of asthmatic symptoms is far better today than it has ever been. Most asthmatics can be cared for out of hospital and can lead full, active lives. The medications available, if used properly, do not have serious long-term problems, nor are they addictive.

In the past, asthmatic attacks were managed either with a gradual build up of medications or none at all. Some regarded the problem as being "all in the child's head" or something that would be "grown out of" and therefore not requiring aggressive treatment. But recent research has shown us that aggressive management of asthma can lead to good results. Asthma should be fought as if it were a fire; it should be "put out" when there are a few sparks, not when there is a raging inferno. Coughing, in most cases, is the earliest warning signal and can be regarded as the sparks and wheezing as the inferno. If the usual asthma medications (as ordered by your doctor) are started when there are only a few "sparks," you may only need to treat your child for a few days. This means he or she can return quickly to school and usual physical activities.

There are certain goals to work towards when treating your child. The medicine must be increased frequently until there is:

- no night or morning coughing
- no coughing (or minimal coughing) with vigorous exercise
- no coughing in cold air
- no coughing with strong smells such as cigarette smoke.

When these goals are achieved the medication can be lowered to maintenance level. If signs of another attack appear, the medication can be increased again. By regulating medications in this way, high dosages may only be needed for short periods of time.

6

Allergic skin diseases

There are three major forms of skin disease caused by allergies:

- eczema
- contact dermatitis
- hives

Eczema

Eczema is a common allergic skin disease in infants. It usually develops when the child is two to six months old and is more common in males than in females.

In most cases, eczema resolves itself in infancy or at least by the time the child is five years old. A few children continue to have eczema after their fifth birthday. One-quarter of these still have the problem as adults and will probably have other allergies as well.

There are two kinds of eczema. **Acute eczema** can make the child very uncomfortable. Red, swollen patches with watery discharge may develop on the skin. However, the problem is relatively short lived. **Chronic eczema** also causes discomfort. It involves scaly, thickened and abnormally dark patches of skin that

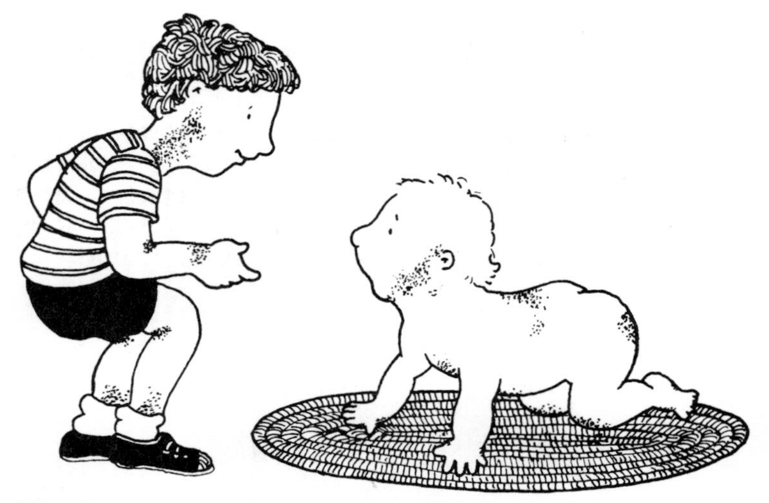

Sites of eczema in children and infants.

crack easily. As its name implies, chronic eczema tends to last, sometimes for years and in rare cases for life.

Areas most often affected by eczema

In infants, eczema usually appears on the cheeks, scalp, neck, back of the arms, front of the legs and trunk. In children over two years old, eczema usually appears in the knee and elbow creases, the neck, wrists and ankles. However, there is overlap between the age groups, and other areas of the body may be involved.

Factors affecting eczema

The exact cause of eczema is not known, but we do know some of the factors that make it develop. One is **climate**. Babies who are brought from warm countries to areas where the climate is cold are particularly vulnerable. Cold, dry air causes the skin to become dry and scaly. The dry, rough areas are easily irritated and become red and itchy. A hot, humid climate which causes sweating tends to make the child scratch the eczema more and hence worsens the rash.

Heredity is also involved. About one-third of children with eczema have parents or other close relatives who have asthma, hay fever or eczema. Just how heredity determines who will have eczema is not known.

Any **skin irritants**, such as rough clothing, soaps, detergents and scratching, can make eczema worse.

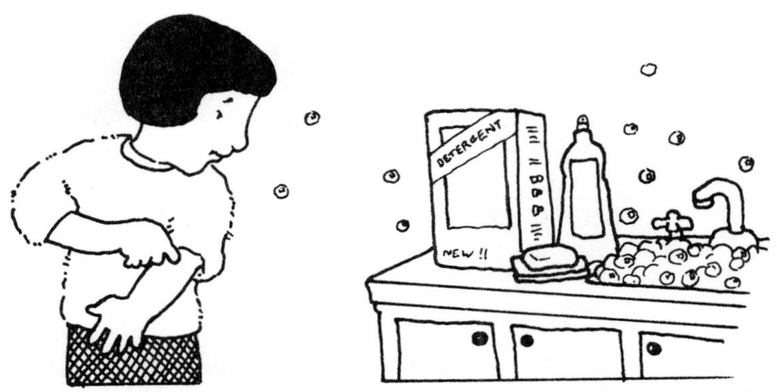

Rough clothing, scratching, harsh soaps and detergents can irritate skin.

Some **foods** cause eczema, especially in babies. Infants who are given cow's milk formula are more likely to have eczema and allergies than those who are breast-fed. Other foods that are most likely to cause problems are eggs, oranges, fish, peanut butter, wheat, pork and chocolate. However, foods are not as frequent a cause of eczema as other factors.

Other ways to help your child

If your child has eczema there are several things you can do to make him or her more comfortable. Since eczema can be a long-term problem, your child may need special care for quite a while. Here are some of the things you can do.

- Keep the temperature in the child's bedroom at 20 °C (68 °F) and the humidity at 30 to 50 per cent.
- Give your child antihistamines to prevent scratching at night.
- Be sure your child's fingernails are kept short so that he or she will not damage the skin with scratching.
- Buy cotton clothing for your child. Certain fabrics, such as wool, silk and nylon, can irritate the skin and make it more difficult to get rid of the eczema.
- Protect your child's skin from cold weather by using oilated creams or emollients at bedtime and before the child goes outside.
- Wash your child's clothes with mild detergent and double rinse the clothes afterwards. (Avoid harsh detergents since they can be irritating.)
- Avoid over-using soaps on the skin during any flare-ups of the eczema and use only mild soaps that are recommended by your physician.
- Frequent bathing may dry the skin and therefore bathing only two to three times a week for short periods of time is recommended. At other times washing the entire body with a damp cloth instead of immersing the child in the bathtub is sufficient.

Treatment of eczema

If your child's eczema has been proven to worsen with milk or other foods, appropriate diets can be prescribed. Avoid random removal of foods from the child's diet for prolonged periods. See page 55 for a more detailed discussion of "elimination diets."

Your doctor will prescribe a treatment appropriate for your child's eczema. For mild cases special creams may be used. These are often applied at least four times a day until the condition improves. For more severe eczema, special baths may be necessary. You may also be advised to use warm mineral oil to remove scales. This process may be followed by an application of prescribed creams. Occasionally drugs are necessary. If there is infection associated with your child's eczema, antibiotics may be needed. Whatever treatment your doctor prescribes, be sure that you follow the instructions you are given carefully and completely.

How easily your child's eczema is controlled depends on various factors. If the eczema is mild, the problem will probably be resolved quickly and easily. Severe cases may take longer. The earlier a doctor diagnoses the eczema and begins treatment the better for your child. Once the causes of your child's eczema are identified, you can minimize exposure to them. This will greatly reduce the severity of the problem.

A few children continue to be bothered by eczema despite treatment. Their eczema may flare up for no apparent reason. Unfortunately, the family may feel it is the child's fault or the parent may feel guilty, suspecting that he or she is doing something wrong. It is important that no one be blamed.

Contact dermatitis

This form of allergic skin disease occurs when a substance irritates the skin by direct contact. Inflammatory changes occur, and as a result the skin has areas of redness with blistering. Eventually a crust forms.

Poison ivy is one of the most common and familiar causes of contact dermatitis. Other leaves such as oak and sumac can also cause dermatitis. The resin in the leaves is the offending agent.

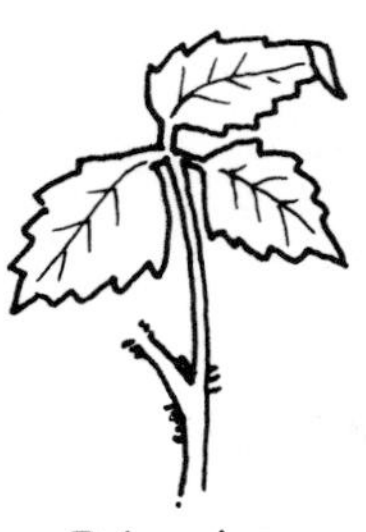
Poison ivy

Other causes of contact dermatitis include cosmetics, soaps, detergents, bubble bath solutions, clothing dyes, paints, chemicals in shoes, rubber and metal products, drugs and medications that are rubbed into the skin.

Diagnosing contact dermatitis

It's usually fairly easy to pinpoint dermatitis. In most cases a rash appears 24 to 48 hours after contact with the offending substance. The skin becomes itchy, red and blisters. Crusts form and last seven to ten days. In difficult-to-diagnose cases, skin tests called patch tests may be used. The offending substance is rubbed onto the skin and covered for 24 to 48 hours.

Treatment of contact dermatitis

Avoiding the irritating substance is the primary form of treatment. Beyond that, medications similar to those used for the treatment of eczema are available. These include antihistamines for itching, special compressing solutions such as Burrows, Cortisone creams and sometimes oral Prednisone. The medications used depend on the severity and the appearance of the rash.

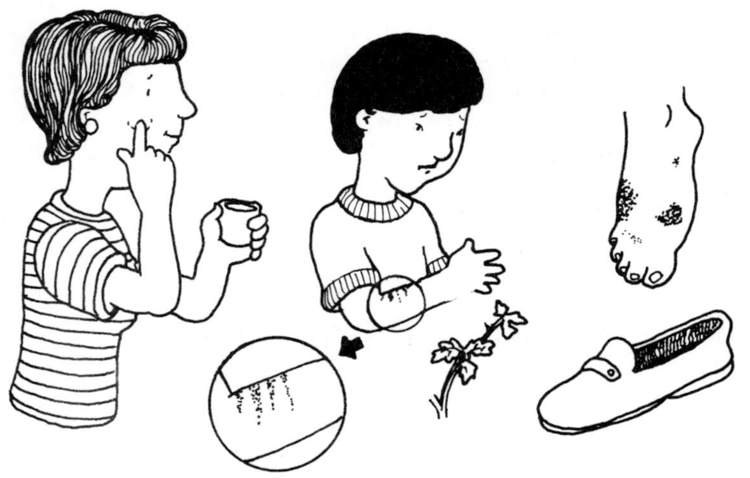

Contact dermatitis can be caused by cosmetics, plants or shoes.

Hives

Hives are itchy skin rashes with red, raised weals of different sizes. Sometimes they look like mosquito bites. They may appear a few at a time or they may be spread over the whole body. Hives come and go and also change places. They last from minutes to days or may recur in crops for a period of weeks or months in different areas. If hives last for more than six weeks they are called **chronic** or **recurrent hives**. Hives lasting less than six weeks are known as **acute** or **sudden onset hives**.

Hives may affect the deeper layers of the skin and cause swelling. This is called angioedema. Hives and angioedema may appear together or separately. Although angioedema can develop anywhere on the body, the areas most commonly affected are the mouth, eyes, tongue, genitals and extremities. Itching may accompany angioedema, but it is not as common as with hives. Sometimes angioedema is painful.

Usually hives disappear without complications. However, if your child develops hives over his or her whole body that rapidly get worse, take him or her to a hospital emergency department or, if your doctor is in, to the doctor's office.

Who do hives affect?

Hives are more common in girls than in boys. They affect children without allergies as well as those with them. Some studies show that over 20 per cent of the population has had hives at some time. Children are more likely to have the acute form of hives, while adults are more likely to have chronic hives, but there is some overlapping.

What causes hives?

Foods: Some foods can cause allergic reactions that involve hives. The most common are milk, eggs, peanuts, berries, fish, shellfish and nuts. Foods and food additives usually cause a sudden onset of hives, but they may also play a role in the more chronic, recurring type of hives.

Drugs: Various drugs, including, among others, penicillin, sulpha, Aspirin, codeine and hormones can cause hives. If a cow is given penicillin for an infection, its milk may contain traces of the drug and become a hidden cause of chronic, recurrent hives. Aspirins in particular can aggravate hives and angioedema. Aspirins should not be given to children who are actively forming hives. Tylenol or Tempra should be used instead for fever or pain. Although the above-mentioned drugs are more commonly involved, any medicine can cause hives in some people. This includes non-prescriptive drugs such as vitamins, laxatives, etc.

If your child has drug allergies be sure your doctor knows about them. It is very important to inform all other doctors who see your child as well. Give the name of the drug and describe your child's reaction to it in detail.

Infections: Hives are associated with numerous infectious diseases including:

- viral infections such as infectious hepatitis and infectious mononucleosis
- fungus infections and parasitic infestations.

Inhaled substances: These include such things as dust, animal danders and pollens. Usually children whose hives are caused by these substances have symptoms of respiratory allergies as well. Other inhalants that may cause hives are aerosols, hair spray, ammonia and cooking odours from foods to which the child is sensitive.

Physical agents: Cold, heat, sunlight, direct pressure, vibration and rubbing the skin may also cause hives in certain children. For example, hives due to cold may occur when the child is exposed to severely cold air or water. The hives may start to appear during exposure to the cold or after the child has entered a warmer area. How these factors cause hives is not fully understood, but treatment *is* available. It is important for the doctor to know exactly what has been happen-

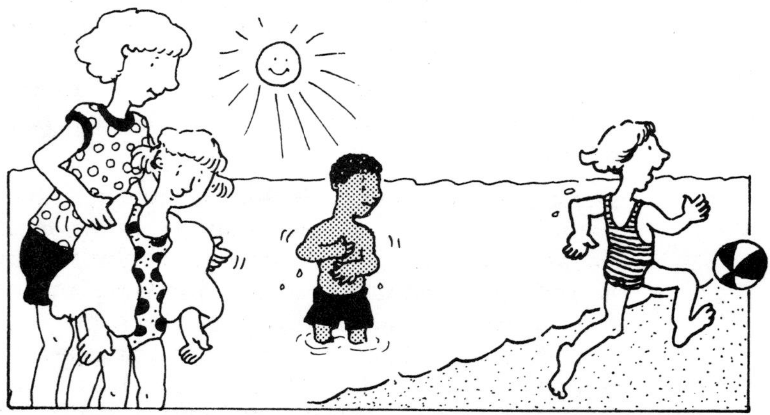

Hives can be caused by rubbing the skin, cold water or excessive heat.

ing to your child. Make sure you observe your child carefully so that you can give the doctor enough information.

Insects: Mosquitos, bed bugs and flea bites can produce small crops of small itchy swellings on exposed parts of the body, especially on the lower extremities in children. These may be a form of hives called papular urticaria. They may clear up in time or with traditional insect bite remedies, but antihistamines will be far more effective.

Psychological factors: Although frequently mentioned, tension and anxiety do not often cause hives. In fact, they may be the *result* of hives. However, psychological factors can make chronic hives worse.

Other causes: Hives can also occur in association with diseases that affect other organs of the body. In this case the hives are not the only abnormality the doctor finds when he or she examines the child.

What you can do

Discovering the exact cause of hives can be extremely difficult. If they occur daily, they are caused by something the child is exposed to frequently. If they seldom occur, they are caused by something the child is not exposed to very often. Sometimes they appear immediately after the offending item is eaten or contacted; at other times it is several hours before the itching begins. Therefore the parent has to act as a detective and try to pinpoint the cause even before seeing the doctor.

If hives last for more than a few days, make a detailed record of everything your child has eaten including drugs and vitamins. List any new or unusual items he or she has been in contact with for the 24 to 48 hour period before the hives developed. Try to observe if the onset of hives is related to the physical agents mentioned earlier. Also make notes on the child's general health and whether he or she has a cold or infection. Because of the complicated nature of the problem it is extremely important to keep a very specific and detailed record. This may help your doctor identify the particular causes of your child's hives.

What the doctor will do

The doctor will first take a history of your child's hives to find what factors are related to the onset of the hives.

Next, the doctor will do a physical examination to determine if the child is suffering from other disease or other allergic reactions elsewhere in his or her body.

Finally, allergy skin tests will be done and possibly some laboratory tests. In many cases allergy testing is not as fruitful in determining the causes of hives as it is for allergic rhinitis.

How hives are treated

Antihistamines are the best treatment for hives. A description of these drugs can be found on page 24. The doctor may have to try two or three different antihistamines to get results and may continue the drug for several days after the hives have disappeared. Occasionally Prednisone tablets may be necessary if the reaction is quite severe.

If the child requires emergency treatment for hives and/or there is associated swelling or breathing difficulty, the doctor may give an epinephrine (adrenalin) injection. After the emergency is over, antihistamines may be prescribed. While hives are present, the child should avoid irritants such as wool clothing, detergents, perfumes, soaps and should not take Aspirin.

Occasionally, if a food is suspected after a history or skin-testing, the food may be eliminated for a short period of time and then reintroduced to see if it is the cause of the hives. For more information on these "elimination diets," see page 55.

How long do hives last?

Usually children have only one episode of hives in their lives. However, if hives recur, the problem may last for a long time. Unless there is an underlying disease, hives do not lead to other problems and will disappear without complications. In the vast majority of children, chronic hives (i.e. hives which recur for more than six weeks) are annoying but not at all harmful.

7

Food allergies

Foods are associated with many problems. They can cause allergic reactions or adverse reactions.

An **allergic food reaction** means that if the child continues to eat the problem food, even in smaller amounts, the reactions will continue and may become more severe. A food allergy reaction may even develop from smelling the food. Food allergies are most common in infancy, and many are outgrown.

An **adverse food reaction** is quite a different problem. It may be heartburn from eating spicy food or stomach pain from eating too many green apples. The same reaction is likely in the future if the same amount of the particular food is eaten. This type of reaction is related to how much of the problem food is eaten. It may not occur at all if very small quantities are eaten. These reactions may persist for life.

Other adverse food reactions occur in those who have enzyme deficiencies which prevent them from digesting certain foods. Children are rarely born with these deficiencies. But they may also develop them after a stomach infection. For example, the enzymes that digest the sugar found in milk, called ''lactose,'' may be destroyed temporarily for days or even months. Milk can then cause problems similar to a true milk allergy such as vomiting, diarrhea and bloating of the

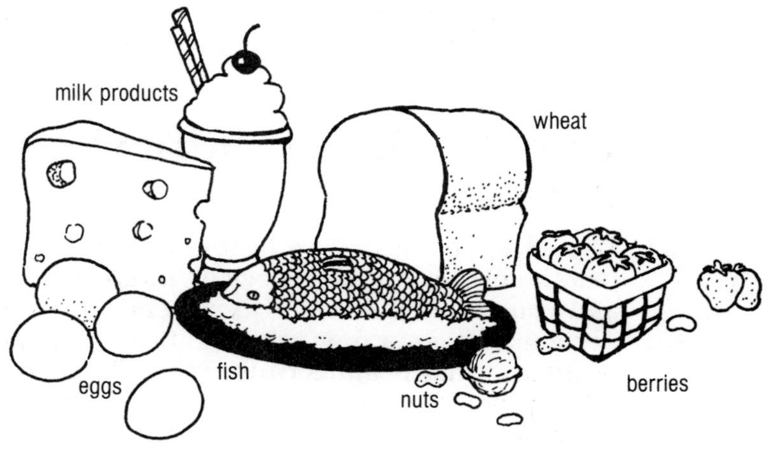

Foods that often cause reactions.

stomach. This problem is usually temporary and of shorter duration than a true milk allergy.

Another common adverse reaction is the association of foods such as chocolate, cheeses and wines with migraine headaches. How foods aggravate a migraine is not completely understood.

The effects of food allergies

People often blame food for problems such as tiredness, paleness, irritability, confusion, nervous tension and bed wetting. But food is unlikely to be responsible in these cases. Such problems may result from various other diseases and should be investigated by a doctor.

Food allergies *are* likely to cause the following:

- gastro-intestinal problems: nausea, vomiting, pain, diarrhea
- skin problems: itching, red rashes, hives
- nose and lung problems: congestion, coughing, wheezing
- life-threatening collapse or shock.

How common are allergies to foods?

No one knows for certain. Many people associate food with problems, but there is no proof that food is to blame. Others eat too much of the wrong foods and then blame the food when they are unwell. The number of proven food allergies is relatively small.

How to identify a food allergy

History

When the doctor takes a history of your child's problem, he or she will be especially interested in what you and your child observed. If your child's lips and face became swollen a few minutes after eating peanuts, it is obvious that peanuts caused the allergic reaction. No other proof is needed. If several hours passed before the reaction developed, it may be more difficult to determine the cause. In this case other factors occurring at the same time could be responsible, including the amount of food eaten, changes in the food produced by cooking, the number of other allergenic foods eaten, other allergic problems and the presence of other illness and environmental factors such as weather changes.

Laboratory tests

If the history fails to show definitely that there is an allergy, skin tests may be used. A drop containing the suspect food is placed on the skin and the skin at the site of the drop is pricked. If redness or significant swelling develops within 20 minutes where the skin was pricked, some reaction has occurred. Whether this indicates an allergy is determined by the size of the reaction. Allergy skin tests are not a perfect guide but they are the best laboratory test available to date. Attempts have been made to develop more accurate blood tests, such as the Rast test, but so far these have not been successful enough to warrant using them in place of skin tests.

Elimination diets

These diets are sometimes used to help identify food allergies. In these diets, suspect food or foods are eliminated and then reintroduced into the diet to see if a reaction occurs. If it does, the food is probably the cause of the allergy.

However, in some elimination diets, *many* foods are removed for *long periods of time*. This may lead to nutritional deficiencies, which are particularly dangerous for allergic children who are frequently ill and need a balanced diet. In addition, behavioural problems can develop when young children are suddenly taken off a wide variety of their favourite foods.

A better approach is to remove only specific suspect foods identified by a history and/or skin testing. Elimination of one food at a time under the guidance of a dietician for a short time, say one to two weeks, and then reintroducing it into the diet when the child is well may help to identify the causative agent.

Another approach, which can be done in a hospital

clinic, is to ''challenge'' the patient with suspect food. To do this, the food is hidden in some other food or juice or made into a powder and given in a capsule. This is done in such a way that the child, parent and doctor do not know what is being given — the so-called double blind technique. This allows for a bias-free observation of any changes in the patient.

One word of caution: foods are not as common a cause of allergic problems as are other factors mentioned in this book. Too much emphasis on diets can distract you from noticing other causes of your child's illness such as weather changes, pollution and so on.

Foods that cause allergic reactions

Any food can cause a reaction in someone. But certain foods do cause problems more frequently than others. These are milk, eggs, wheat, fish, nuts and berries.

Variations in food reactions

Children who react to certain foods may not always have a problem with that food. Their reaction may have been caused by the way the food was prepared, how much was eaten and so on. It is obviously helpful to identify these variations so that appropriate precautions can be taken.

Some foods, such as eggs or milk, may cause problems when they are eaten uncooked but do not cause problems if they are eaten cooked. In this case, the cooking destroys the element in the food that causes the allergic reaction.

Sometimes people do not have reactions to a particular food if they eat it only occasionally. If they change their eating habits and begin to eat the food frequently, problems will result. This type of diet change often occurs when particular fruits are in season.

The age of the child also affects food allergies. Infants and children are more likely to have reactions to foods than adults. Very young children cannot digest food completely and therefore their bodies absorb the whole proteins. When whole proteins are absorbed they are more likely to cause problems. Although many food allergies are primarily associated with infancy and childhood, others may remain for life; these include allergies to peanuts and shellfish.

In some cases, sensitivity to a particular food *increases* with age. Over the years, a person may become so sensitive that he or she is apt to have a violent reaction from simply smelling the food (e.g. eggs, fish) cooking.

Other tips

The plants we eat can be divided into food families. Knowing this may be important. If a child has an allergy to one item in a family of foods, other foods in the same family may cause problems too. Some food families are:

- peanuts belong to the pea family
- potatoes and tomatoes belong to the nightshade family
- almonds belong to the plum family
- melons, cucumbers, squash and pumpkins belong to the gourd family.

Sensitivity to one form of animal protein does not necessarily mean sensitivity to another form. For example, children who are allergic to milk may be able to eat beef or inhale cattle dander without problems. Children who are allergic to eggs may not be allergic to the meat or feathers of chickens. The opposite is also possible.

Food additives

Thousands of food additives are used in preparing foods to ensure their safety and quality when they reach the consumer's table. We cannot do without these additives because of the way the food is produced and distributed. However, some additives may cause problems for some children.

To date, we only have a limited understanding of the effects of food additives. They have been suspected in many allergic problems, such as wheezing, nasal stuffiness and hives. But there are no skin or blood tests that can help us discover whether these substances are actually causing allergies. Only by removing them from the diet and then adding them again can reactions be determined.

Additives are found in almost every food, so it is impossible to eliminate them completely. However, the consumption of foods that contain large amounts of additives can be reduced. Such foods are soft drinks, candies, bakery goods, cereals, ice cream, sherbet, salad dressings, jams, jellies, prepared gravies, sauces, ketchup and spices. These foods if eaten in excess are not nutritionally adequate, hence avoiding them will not impair a child's diet. Eating a nutritionally sound diet will allow your child to avoid large doses of additives.

Chemicals in foods

Natural

Natural toxins such as myristicin (a hallucinogen found in nutmeg and carrots), nitrates (a carcinogen found in lettuce and celery) and solanine (a nerve poison found in potatoes) are found in extremely small amounts so they are not a concern.

Artificial

Additives are used to enhance the colour, flavour and stability of food products. Included are food colourings, flavouring agents, preservatives and emulsifiers, stabilizers, thickening agents, firming agents and many more.

Food colouring agents include such compounds as tartrazine yellow dye #5 and erythrosine red dye #3. In Canada there are six major dyes and several minor dyes. They are found in the following foods: soft drinks, candies, dessert powders, snack foods, bakery goods, dried cereals, salad dressings, gravies, nuts and spices, jams and jellies, food packaging materials, ice cream, sherbets, butter, cheese, maraschino cherries and sausage casings. Foods such as bread, meat, potatoes, fruit and milk fluid products do not contain these dyes. Tartrazine has been incriminated in asthma, nasal stuffiness and hives. But recent research shows that this problem may not be as common as previously believed.

Food flavourings are found naturally as well. For ex-

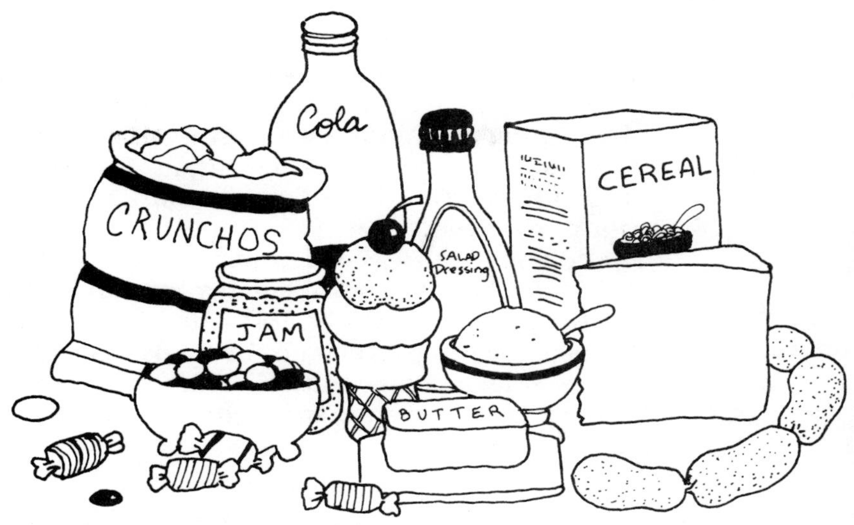

Foods that often contain food dyes.

ample, an apple alone has 80 different chemical components. Fortunately many of these natural food flavourings have not been shown to cause problems. However, flavour enhancers such as monosodium glutamate have been shown to cause problems such as wheezing and the "Chinese food restaurant syndrome," which is a feeling of tightness in the chest, rapid heartbeat, flushing and headache after eating chinese food that contains this additive.

Food preservatives include benzoates, BHA (butylated hydrozyanisole), BHT (butylated hydrotoluene) and sulfites. All of these produce asthma. But with the exception of sulfites, the problem is not as serious as people once thought it to be. Benzoates are found in jams and jellies, mincemeat, marmalades, ketchup, marinated meat and fish and some fruits such as prunes, plums, cranberries and loganberries. BHA and BHT are found in vegetable oils and shortening, dry breakfast cereals, beverage mixes, chewing gum, potato chips, instant potatoes and margarine.

Sulfites have recently been found to be a cause of significant wheezing. They can produce a severe attack in 5 to 10 per cent of asthmatics. They are found in many foods such as dehydrated fruits and vegetables, marmalades, ketchup, molasses, frozen mushrooms, manufactured meats and sausages, fruit juices, soft drinks, wines, beers, cider and vinegar. Foods eaten at home do not contain high enough levels to cause harm.

But restaurant foods such as salad bar ingredients, avocado dips, wines and beers are high in sulfites. Since severe attacks have been reported within 30 minutes after eating restaurant meals, asthmatics should inquire if sulfites are used by the restaurant. Fortunately legislation to remove sulfites from restaurants is being currently reviewed.

Additives are a necessary part of both food manufacturing and distribution. While concern about them is justified, there is no need for panic about them. A well-balanced diet and avoidance of foods that contain additives in high concentrations, such as non-nutritious foods or certain restaurant foods, is more than adequate protection.

Food allergies and hyperactivity

About ten years ago, Dr. Ben Feingold made headlines by suggesting that there were strong links between additives and hyperactivity. More recently sugar has been implicated as well. And some studies even suggest that foods such as wheat or milk are to blame. Studies in the United States and Canada over the past decade and our experience at the Hospital for Sick Children do not support these theories. To date, a consistent connection between hyperactivity and foods has not been proven. In fact several Canadian studies have shown that sugar, rather than causing undesirable behaviour in the hyperactive or normal child, may even produce a calming or sedating effect.

We believe that a child who is eating a well-balanced diet is not likely to have a problem with sugar. Children who have allergic reactions over a long period of time may become irritable and hyperactive perhaps because of lack of sleep or other factors. The hyperactive behaviour is not necessarily linked to a food. However, if you still feel a particular food is causing a problem, your doctor should be able to help sort it out.

Physical problems such as hearing impairment can also lead to hyperactive behaviour. Therefore a complete physical should be your first step if you feel that your child is hyperactive. In addition you should also take note of when the hyperactive behaviour occurs. Sometimes in young children, changes in their daily routine such as a lengthy visit to a relative's home, shopping trips or prolonged car rides may bring on hyperactivity rather than the foods eaten at those times.

Treatment of food allergies

The only treatment for a food allergy is to avoid the problem food. If the allergy is caused by such common items as milk, wheat or eggs, it will be necessary to get a special diet from your doctor. Even with a special diet, you should read all food labels carefully.

Infants may ''grow out of'' food allergies as they get older. With your doctor's permission you can challenge your child by giving him or her the problem food every three to six months. When the child no longer reacts to the food he or she has outgrown the allergy.

Allergies to some foods (e.g., nuts, shellfish) appear to last for many years. In these cases the child should continue to avoid them. Rechallenging should not be done unless advised by a doctor.

Can food allergies be prevented?

Babies born to families with a strong history of food and/or other allergies are likely to have problems in infancy and early childhood. Such babies should be breast-fed or given a soybean formula such as Prosobee, Isomil or Soyalac. Appropriate feeding will not prevent allergies, but it may delay or modify their development in the early months of life. When the mother is breast-feeding an infant who is likely to have allergies, she should avoid excessive amounts of cow's milk or other highly allergenic foods such as wheat, since these could cause problems for her baby. Introduction of allergenic foods can be done near the end of the first year.

Researchers are now experimenting with new drugs that can be taken orally to prevent allergic food reactions. These would be especially useful for children with multiple food allergies for whom it is difficult to plan a nutritious diet.

8

Drug reactions

A drug reaction is a sometimes harmful reaction that is not related to the normal action of the drug. In other words, it is not like a side effect which, although unpleasant, is anticipated because of the way the drug works.

Most reactions to drugs are not allergic in nature because they do not involve an allergen-antibody reaction. How they work is not fully understood.

But some drugs *do* cause allergic reactions, most notably penicillin. Sensitivity can develop anywhere from a few minutes to a few days. Once a child has become sensitized to penicillin he or she may remain sensitized to it for a long time and will have an immediate reaction even to very small doses of the drug.

If your child has a known drug allergy and the drug is avoided, a reaction is still possible because drugs can be taken in hidden forms. For example, milk from a cow that had been given penicillin could contain the drug and affect your child.

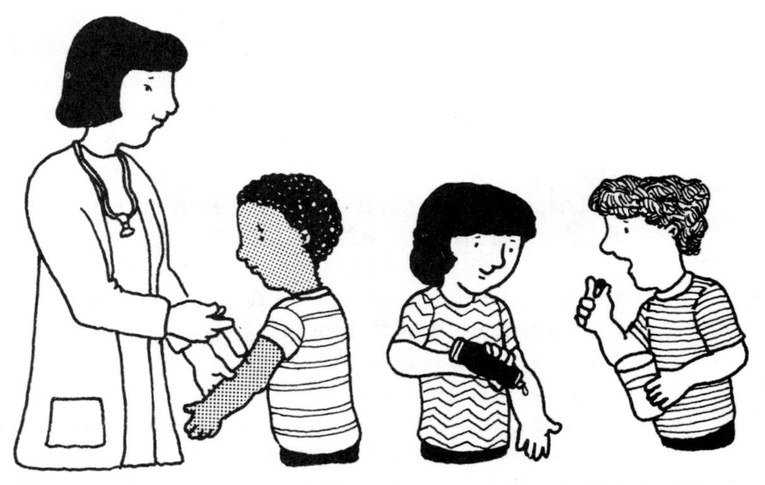

Drug reactions can occur when drugs are injected, applied to the skin or swallowed.

Which drugs cause reactions?

Any drug can cause an adverse reaction, even many non-prescription medications. A reaction may occur regardless of the way the drug is used, that is whether it is applied to the skin as a cream or swallowed as a tablet. Items that one might not think of as drugs, including Aspirins and vitamins, can also cause drug reactions.

Some common causes of drug reactions are alcohol, antibiotics (including penicillin, sulpha, tetracycline), anticonvulsants, Aspirin, bromides, hormones (including insulin), iodides, laxatives, local anaesthetics, narcotics (including codeine, morphine), sedatives (including phenobarbital), tranquillizers, vaccines and vitamins.

How common are adverse drug reactions?

Anyone can develop an adverse reaction to a drug. However, only about one-quarter of drug reactions involve allergic sensitization.

Allergy to penicillin is common whether or not one has other allergies. The fact that there is no family history of allergic disease is no guarantee that a person will not react to the drug.

Recognizing an adverse drug reaction

If your child becomes sensitized to a drug it is important to recognize what is happening. Reactions can vary in severity and type. Some require immediate attention; none should be ignored.

Skin reactions involve itching, hives or rashes all over the body. They can be made worse by exposure to the sun.

Respiratory (breathing) reactions involve rhinitis or an inflammation of the mucus membrane of the nose. The child might suddenly seem to have a cold or hay fever. A drug allergy could also cause an asthma attack.

Severe drug reactions can cause the child to collapse and go into shock.

What to do

1. Stop giving the child the drug.
2. Consult your doctor.
3. If the reaction is severe, get medical help immediately. Take your child to a hospital emergency department or, if the doctor is in his or her office, to your doctor.
4. Keep a permanent record of the exact drug prescribed and the reactions your child had.

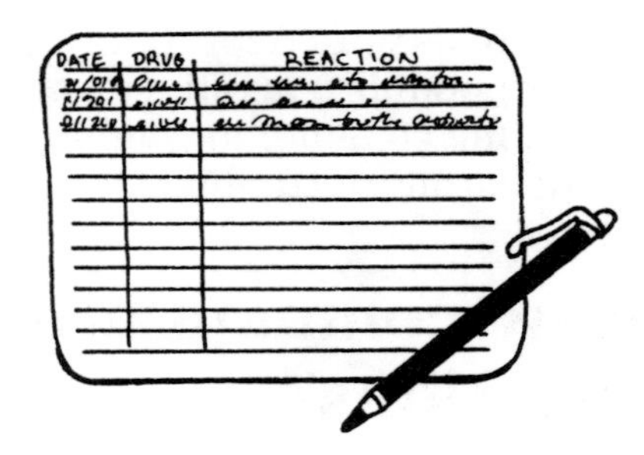

Identifying adverse drug reactions

History

The doctor must have an accurate history of what drugs were taken and exactly what symptoms the child had after taking them. Without these details he or she cannot pinpoint a drug reaction problem.

Tests

Very few tests are currently available to diagnose adverse drug reactions. Penicillin allergy is one of the few sensitivities that *can* be reliably confirmed by skin testing. The skin tests, however, are not routinely available and should be primarily used if penicillin must be given. If the various skin tests for penicillin are negative, the risk of reaction is the same as in the general population. However, if the penicillin skin tests are positive, and the individual is then given penicillin, more than 50 per cent will have a reaction.

New or more effective blood tests such as antibody detection tests are constantly being developed for drug sensitivity. However, there is as yet no reliable method of identifying drug allergies from a blood sample.

The drug can also be given orally or by injection and the child can be monitored for a reaction. This is called challenge testing, and it is only done in a hospital under the doctor's control. It is also only undertaken if the drug is to be given immediately after the testing has been done. This latter method can be used for other drugs as well as penicillin. However, it is a crude technique, and the results do not guarantee freedom from problems in future. Hence this type of test might have to be done each time the drug is required.

Treatment of adverse drug reactions

Treatment of drug reactions varies with the severity of the problem. In all cases, however, the offending drug is stopped and should not be taken again.

Treatment of skin reactions

The doctor may prescribe medication for your child to take orally and/or preparations to be used on the skin. Antihistamines are often prescribed in cases of hives, and corticosteroids may be used if the problem does not clear up readily. Usually medication is not required for more than two weeks.

Special bath preparations may be used. For example, your child may have to soak twice a day in a bath containing Oilated Aveeno. Until the skin problem clears, the child may also have to use a mild soap such as an Aveeno Bar or Dove soap and lubricating oils such as Alpha-Keri.

Harsh fabrics such as wool or starched linen should not be worn, and sunlight should be avoided as much as possible.

Treatment of severe reactions

Severe reactions require immediate medical care. The doctor will give an injection of adrenalin, ensure that the child's airways are kept open, provide oxygen as needed and give intravenous fluid therapy.

Precautions the doctor will take

1. Your doctor will not prescribe any drug that has previously caused a reaction in your child or drugs that are chemically related to the drug in question.
2. Synthetically produced drugs will be substituted for organically produced hormones where possible.
3. Your doctor will try to give your child drugs that are prepared with a minimum of preservatives or colouring.
4. If your child is allergic to eggs, tell your doctor. He or she may want to test your child's sensitivity to vaccines containing eggs. Your doctor may refer the child to an allergist for this procedure.

If your child has had a drug reaction

1. **Read labels carefully**. Do not give your child any preparation containing the drug that causes the reaction.
2. Be sure your doctor knows all the details about the allergy.
3. Consider providing your child with a Medic-Alert bracelet to wear all the time. These can be obtained from: Canadian Medic-Alert Foundation, 293 Eglinton Ave. E., Toronto, Ontario M4P 2Z8, Telephone (416) 481-5175.

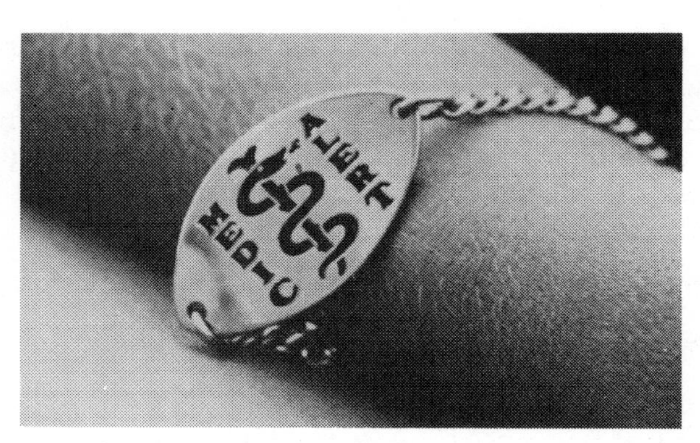

Hidden hazards in drugs

All drugs, whether pills or liquids, have additives such as binders, colourings, flavouring or sweetening agents, lubricants and preservatives. These help the medicine dissolve faster, taste better and stay fresher. However, they can also cause reactions. Many patients who appear to be reacting to unrelated drugs may be reacting instead to a common additive or preservative in these drugs. The task of identifying the cause of these reactions is difficult. It is made even more difficult in Canada because many of the agents are not listed on the drug packages or bottles. The United States now has legislation that requires complete labelling of all agents used in the preparation of the drugs. However, this is not yet required in Canada.

Accessibility to this information would facilitate doctors' attempts to identify problem agents and enable research workers to determine whether or not these additives are indeed causing significant adverse reactions.

9

Allergies to stinging insects

Allergic reactions to insect bites have been known since ancient times. The first recorded reaction to a wasp sting involved an Egyptian Pharoah who was stung around 2800 B.C.

The four types of stinging insects in North America are:

- mosquitos
- flies, including deer flies and black flies
- hymenoptera family, including bees, hornets, wasps and yellow jackets
- fire ants (found around the Gulf of Mexico and New Orleans).

There are two types of reaction to insect bites. One is a **local reaction** which affects the skin where the bite occurred. The other is a **general**, or **anaphylactic**, **reaction** which can affect the whole body and may be life-threatening. Most people have local reactions.

Local reactions

Local reactions are usually short lived. There may be discomfort or pain for a few hours and swelling is common. The swelling may occur immediately after the bite or one to two days later. It may be very large, sometimes the size of a small grapefruit. It may last for a few days but usually disappears on its own.

How to treat local reactions

The first step in dealing with a local reaction is to decide whether the insect left its stinger in the child's skin. Honey bees have barbed stingers that stay in the skin and continue to pump more venom. If the child was stung by a bee, you should remove the stinger immediately with tweezers or your fingernails. Try not to squeeze the stinger because that releases more venom into the child. Other insects of the hymenoptera group such as hornets, wasps and yellow jackets do not leave their stingers behind.

Calamine lotion and ice packs may be used to relieve itching and pain. Sometimes oral antihistamines are used to relieve itching. Scratching with dirty hands or fingernails could lead to infection, so advise your child not to scratch.

General (anaphylactic) reactions

General reactions are not common but they can be serious. When they occur within a few seconds to an hour after the bite they are called anaphylactic reactions.

The symptoms of general reactions are:

- itchiness and hives over the whole body
- nausea, vomiting, diarrhea
- lightheadedness
- swelling of the eyelids, lips or tongue
- difficulty breathing
- rapid heart beat
- loss of consciousness or seizures.

How to treat a general reaction

If your child has a general reaction after being stung by an insect, take him or her to a doctor immediately. Although very few people die (for example, only two in Ontario between 1970 and 1975), a fatal reaction is possible if appropriate treatment is not given.

Once a child has had a general reaction, you should make sure you have medication to use in case of another sting. Available kits, called ANA Kits, contain a preloaded adrenalin injection, an antihistamine and a tourniquet. Premeasured adrenalin doses are also available in injecting devices called EpiPens. Your doctor will explain how to use them and what dose of the medicine to use. Kits should be kept at home, in the car, at cottages — anywhere a sting is possible.

Your child should also wear a Medic-Alert bracelet to indicate a sensitivity to insects. These can be obtained from: Canadian Medic-Alert Foundation, 293 Eglinton Ave. E., Toronto, Ontario M4P 2Z8, Telephone (416) 481-5175.

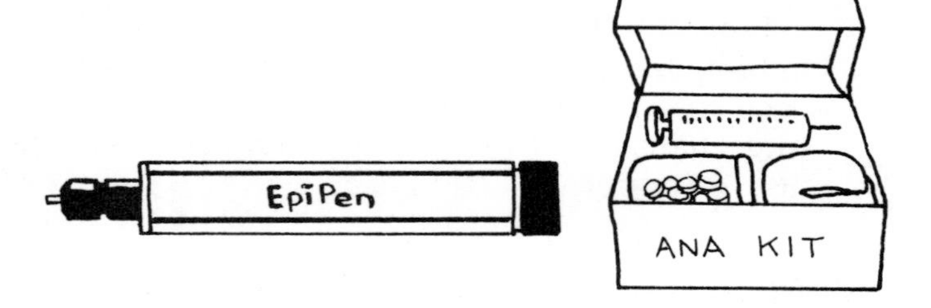

Prevention of future attacks

The possibility of increasing your child's tolerance to insect stings should be discussed with your doctor. This procedure, known as immunotherapy or hyposensitization, is done by using injections of insect venom. At present it is used only for reactions to the hymenoptera group and not for mosquitoes or flies.

Immunotherapy, or allergy shots, for bee stings is currently recommended when there is a history of general reactions involving breathing difficulty or loss of consciousness. It is *not* recommended for itchiness or hives resulting from a sting. It is not yet known how long these injections must be given. Immunotherapy does not lessen the need to practise the commonsense rules that follow for avoiding insect stings.

How to avoid insect stings

Explain to your child where stinging insects are likely to be:

- **Honeybees** live in hives in old trees and are often found in clover.
- **Wasps** nest in sheltered places, such as the eaves of buildings, behind shutters, shrubs and woodpiles.
- **Hornets** nest in bushes or high in trees.
- **Yellow jackets** nest under logs or rocks or in the ground and may emerge through a small hole in the ground.

Also be sure that your child is aware of, and obeys, the following rules for dealing safely with stinging insects.

1. Do not walk barefoot or wear open-toed sandals anywhere. Even hard beach sand can harbour cer-

tain types of wasps.

2. Do not use perfumes, hairsprays, hair tonics or other cosmetics as these may attract insects.
3. Avoid loose clothing in which insects may become trapped.
4. Avoid brightly coloured clothing or clothes made from rough materials such as corduroy or denim since these can attract insects.
5. Avoid keeping food, especially highly sugared food, outside unless it is properly covered.
6. Avoid outdoor trash cans as these often attract insects.
7. Do not touch objects outside without first looking to see whether there is an insect on or in them.
8. Do not idly kick rotting logs or bushes that are unfamiliar to you.
9. Do any gardening cautiously to avoid striking a hidden nest.
10. If a bee lands on you, do not slap it. Instead, gently blow it away.
11. Try using insect repellants. (Unfortunately, these are often of little use.)

As a parent you can help by:

- Keeping the area around garbage cans clean and occasionally spraying the area with insecticide.
- If a bee or a wasp hitches a ride in your car, open all windows and it will leave. Panic may cause an accident.
- Have nests and hives around your home removed by a professional exterminator or by someone who is not insect sensitive.

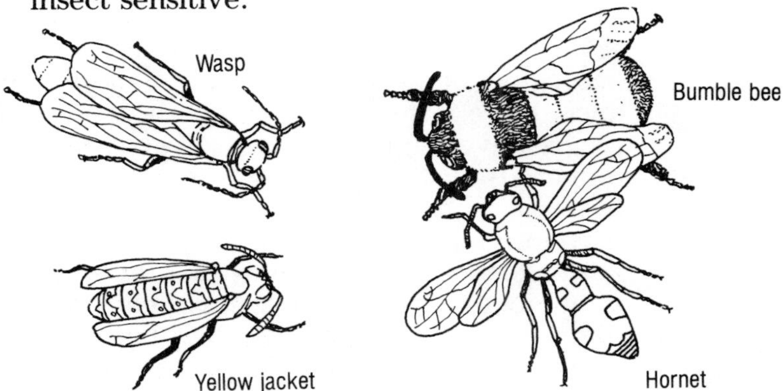

10

Coping with the environment

If a child suddenly develops allergies, your family doctor or allergy specialist may suggest making changes in the child's environment — your home. People sometimes feel that changes are not necessary because the child has been exposed to the home surrounding all of his or her life and hasn't been bothered previously. But this is not the case.

When a child starts to have allergy problems it is as if a light switch went on in his or her body. He or she now becomes sensitive to many things in the environment that did not cause problems before. You may have experienced this for yourself. For example, cigarette smoke may not normally bother you. But if you have a cold, smoke may make you feel unpleasantly stuffed up. It is as if the cold had turned on a switch in your body, making you more sensitive to smoke.

The same thing happens in an allergic child. If the child develops an allergy to, say, cats, he or she becomes switched on to other potential allergens, such as dust, or irritants, such as pollution.

Once this switch is turned on for an allergic child, he or she is more likely to experience problems. This means, for example, that the longer your child is exposed to a potential allergy cause, such as dust, the more likely he or she is to become allergic to it.

How many changes are needed?

The changes you need to make are determined by the severity of your child's illness. If allergic reactions occur only occasionally and are no more than a nuisance, there is no need to go overboard and, for example, remove the family pet. However, if the child is on numerous medications and/or is admitted frequently to hospital, more changes will be necessary. Or if a child is born into a family where there are numerous people with allergies, it is definitely helpful to arrange the environment as if the child were already allergic. This will not completely prevent allergies, but it may lessen the severity of the reactions and it is especially important for infants, who are more vulnerable than the older child. Many of the changes suggested in the following sections can be accomplished without giving the child the feeling that he or she is isolated or in some way handicapped.

A conservative approach

Allergists believe in a conservative approach to changing the environment. Clinical ecologists, on the other hand, advocate a much more radical approach. They believe that stresses on the body such as exposure to toxic chemicals, even at low levels, over a prolonged period of time may prove harmful. They maintain that there are many such chemicals; those posing the greatest hazard, they believe, are carbon monoxide from gas stoves, furnaces and heaters, nitrogen dioxide from tobacco smoke and indoor combustion, formaldehyde from building materials and furnishings and radon gas in homes with poor ventilation. Even normally benign items such as soft plastic materials are felt to give off irritating fumes.

Scientific studies have not been able to incriminate these chemicals and others like them. Most studies have shown that they have minimal direct effect on peoples' allergies. Therefore, at present, the need to "strip one's house" completely, install expensive filtration systems, repaint and so on is open to question. There is no doubt, however, that defects in house construction or in heating, cooling or ventilation systems that allow high levels of irritants or chemicals to build up have to be corrected. There is a definite need for more detailed research in this area. In the meantime, changes that are made should be based on a sound scientific evaluation, especially before incurring massive expenses.

Identifying problem areas

Keeping a diary of your child's symptoms might help you answer the following questions:

- Are symptoms worse inside the home?
- Are they worse in a certain room?
- Do symptoms get better when the furnace is off or the windows open?

- Did the symptoms change when you moved or have recent changes been made to the house, such as insulating, remodelling or purchasing new appliances?
- Are there any unusual smells?
- Are there damp areas?
- Is the house very old?
- Are symptoms better out of the house or on vacation?
- Do symptoms disappear if you discontinue any hobbies in the house, for example, those using glues, paints, etc.?

What changes are necessary?

We have divided the changes needed into the following sections:

- House dust control
- Mould elimination
- Animals and birds
- Pollens
- Indoor air pollution and tobacco smoke
- Workplace irritants in the home
- Unusual plant allergies
- Mechanical devices for environmental control

It is important to realize that all sections may apply to your child — either now or in the future. Although it may not be necessary to make all of the changes suggested in all of the sections, small changes in each section may add up to a significant benefit. Again, the changes you must make depend on the severity of your child's problem.

House dust control

House dust is a complex mixture of many different particles such as mould, fungi, animal products, debris from furniture, food remnants, insect parts and outdoor dust. One of the major components, and a specific cause of problems, is the house dust mite, a microscopic creature which survives in dust best when the temperature is 25 °C (77 °F) and the humidity is greater than 60 per cent. These creatures seem to prefer mattresses, carpeting and upholstered furniture.

The following suggestions are directed towards dust

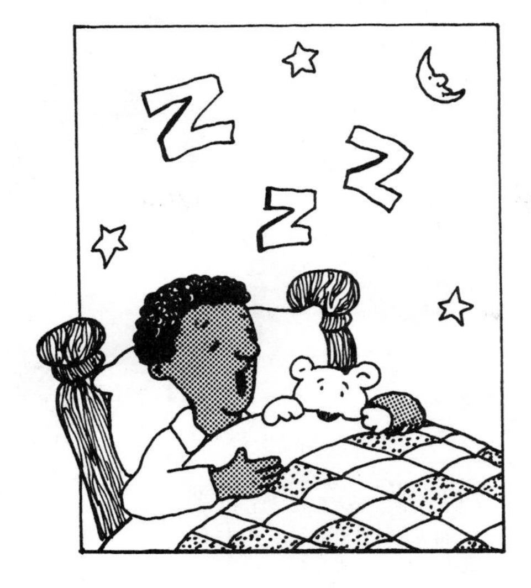

control in your child's **bedroom**. Since a third of the day is spent in the bedroom, it makes sense to concentrate on this room. Many of these suggestions can be used in other parts of your house too, especially in areas where your child spends a lot of time.

Floors

Bare wood or linoleum floors are best. Avoid wool or shag carpets. If the child wants a rug near the bed, choose a small washable one. Underpads should be made of foam.

If your child's room already has wall-to-wall carpeting, vacuum the whole floor every week. Have the carpet steam-cleaned once or twice a year. Using rug shampoos is not sufficient; they do not remove deeply imbedded dust particles.

Windows

Keep the inside of the windows clean. Use short, light curtains that are made of smooth, washable cotton or polyester (Dacron, Terylene, etc.). Use roll-up window blinds. Avoid dust-collecting venetian blinds and shutters.

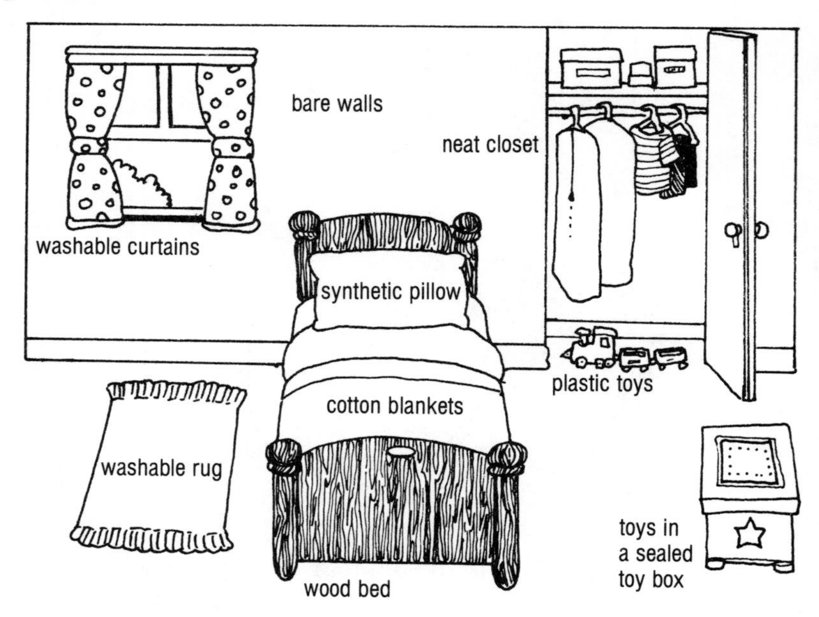

Furniture

Furniture made from wood, plastic or vinyl is preferable. Do not use upholstered or over-stuffed furniture because it collects dust. Avoid old leather furniture because it may collect mould.

All beds in the allergic child's room must be made up in the same way. Do not put canopies over beds. If you have bunk beds, give the top bed to the child who has allergies. Better still, convert bunk beds into twin beds. The bed used by the allergic child should be placed so that it is not in the direct line of any air vent that could blow dust onto him or her.

Completely wrap the mattress and box spring with plastic or vinyl covers. These covers should be zippered or taped closed and checked regularly for cracks. Replace them whenever holes or cracks appear. Vacuum both the mattress and the box spring every time you change the bed. Mattresses and box springs more than ten years old should probably be discarded.

Bedding

All bedding must be washable. Use synthetic or cotton blankets and bedspreads and wash them regularly. Use a polyester mattress pad or several sheets doubled over.

This is especially important if your child has skin reactions because it will prevent the plastic mattress cover from causing sweating and irritating the skin.

Use synthetic pillows. Do not use pillows stuffed with kapok, feathers or down. Foam rubber pillows should be cleaned regularly because they may collect moulds.

Walls and ceiling

Walls and ceiling should be painted or covered with wallpaper that can be washed easily. Avoid all dust-collecting items such as rugs, pennants, chalkboards, open shelves, hanging plants, mobiles, etc.

Closets

Avoid storing clothing for several seasons in the closet. If clothes must be stored in the closet, put them in tightly zippered garment bags. Do not store sports equipment or other dust-collecting items in the closet. Avoid mothballs and other chemicals. Keep the closet door closed whenever possible.

Toys

Toys left sitting around in the bedroom will collect dust. Be sure your child has toys that can be washed easily. Fuzzy or stuffed toys that are not machine washable should be avoided. Instead choose toys made from plastic, metal or wood. Keep toys in a closed box, drawer or cabinet. If your home has a playroom, keep all the toys there.

Clutter

Minimize clutter. Keep books, toys and sports equipment put away in bookcases, boxes or drawers when they are not in use. If they are seldom used, store them somewhere other than in the allergic child's bedroom.

Cleaning

Keep the allergic child away from the room when

cleaning is being done. Clean the room by wet mopping and dusting at least twice a week and possibly every day during the allergy season. Water is the best cleaning agent and should be used instead of spray cleaners and waxes that could irritate the child. Do not use brooms and dry dusters; these tend to spread dust around instead of removing it.

Once a month, wash the entire room, including the baseboards and the floor under the furniture. Also once a month, wash all bedding (including the pillows, mattress cover, bedspread and blankets) and curtains whenever possible, dry the bedding and any other laundry in an automatic dryer. Do not leave freshly washed bedding and clothes on outdoor clotheslines any longer than necessary to dry them. Otherwise dust and pollen will collect on them.

Vacuum non-washable items such as wall-to-wall carpeting regularly. Be sure to take the vacuum cleaner outside before removing the dust bag.

When the cleaning is finished, close the windows and doors for an hour or two before your child goes into the room.

Other tips

Keep the doors and windows in your child's bedroom closed as much as possible. Do not allow drafts or cross ventilation. If you want to air the room, do so when the child is not in the room or during the middle of the day, when the pollen count is lowest.

Regardless of the exact nature of fabrics used, all rugs, bedding and furniture stuffings in the home may become a problem after prolonged use and aging.

Mould elimination

Moulds or mildews are types of fungus. They live off decaying plant life. Moulds give off spores which become airborne. The air is never free of spores. When they are inhaled by a sensitive person, they can produce allergic symptoms. Moulds in the home are found all year round; those in the soil are found from spring to fall.

How to avoid moulds

Moulds are associated with dampness or high humidity. Here are some situations in which moulds are likely to be present. A mould-sensitive person should avoid these situations or at least reduce his or her exposure to them.

Outdoor moulds can be encountered:

- cutting grass
- raking or burning leaves
- making compost piles
- harvesting grain
- cutting or binding hay
- hiking in forests or woods, especially near piles of fallen leaves or rotting wood
- in farms or barns that have hay or other grains stored in them or damp sheds or garages
- in cottages, hotels and motels, especially when they are first opened for the season
- during warm humid weather which allows optimum growth of moulds
- during hot, dry, windy weather which helps disperse the moulds in the air.

Indoor moulds are often found in:

- unfinished basements, crawl spaces and attics
- shower stalls, cracks between bathroom tiles, refrigerator drip trays, window mouldings, garbage bins, utility rooms
- aquariums
- dried flowers and potted plants
- air conditioners, dehumidifiers, humidifiers and vaporizers that are not cleaned every week
- furnace filters that are not changed regularly
- camping equipment (sleeping bags, boat cushions, etc.)
- old foam rubber pillows or mattresses
- damp closets or closets in which damp shoes and clothing have been placed
- leather goods
- surfaces soiled by children or pets
- stored foods such as dried fruit, vegetables, bread, cheese
- liquids such as beer, wine, vinegar and soya sauce.

How to reduce indoor moulds

- Control house dust (see page 74).
- Wash surfaces such as window ledges and shower stalls with Lysol or chlorine bleach at least once every three months.
- Use mould-resistant paints on walls in unfinished basements.
- Use dehumidifiers in unfinished or damp basements in humid weather.
- Clean equipment such as furnace filters, air conditioners, dehumidifiers, humidifiers and vaporizers frequently.
- Minimize the number of house plants or cover the soil with aluminum foil. If possible, use mould-inhibiting solutions in the soil. These can be obtained from local nurseries.
- Cover the ground in crawl spaces with black polyethylene sheets to reduce moisture.
- Install effective drains to remove standing water in crawl spaces.

Animals and birds

Animals and birds have dander (skin scales) or feathers that may cause allergies. There are no "non-allergenic" animals. Small, non-shedding animals may cause allergies just as larger, longer haired animals do because it is dander, not hair, which causes the problem. A sensitive child may even have a reaction to urine from guinea pigs and saliva from dogs or cats.

Removing the animal from your home may be necessary. Even then, since the dander and feathers may become airborne, it may take three to six months after the animal is gone for the irritants to disappear completely.

If you cannot part with your animal follow these rules:

- Never allow the animal into the allergic child's bedroom.
- Do not allow the child to wash the animal, especially indoors.
- Keep the animal outside as much as possible.
- Do not replace pets that die and do not add any new pets to your home. Skin tests may show that a child is

allergic to only one species of dog or cat or other pet. This does not mean that the child can safely be exposed to other types of animals. If a child that is allergic to one kind of animal is exposed to another kind, he or she may become sensitized to that animal too.

- Encourage other family members who have close contact with an animal elsewhere to change their clothes when they enter the house.
- Request that babysitters who have animals in their homes wear clothes that have had little or no contact with their animals when they look after your child.
- Before you visit in a home where there is an animal, give your child antihistamines or anti-asthma medication so that he or she can tolerate limited exposure to the animal. If the child is to stay overnight, the animal should be temporarily removed. The room the child occupies should be cleaned thoroughly and the bedding should be changed before the visit.
- When camping, do not let your pet sleep in the same tent or cabin as the allergic child and do not travel with the child and the animal in the same vehicle.
- Make an effort to keep all animals that are known to cause allergies out of your child's classroom at school.

Other tips

- Children who are allergic to feathers should avoid contact with live birds but can eat the meat from chickens, turkeys and other fowl.
- Children who are allergic to fish may also be sensitive to glue since some glues, such as LePage's, are derived from fish.
- Children who are allergic to animals can usually wear clothes made from processed wool. However, since these clothes may collect dust they must be washed or cleaned frequently to avoid irritating.

Pollens

Pollens are the fertilizing agent of flowering plants, including trees, grass and weeds. Some flowers, such as goldenrod and roses, have sticky pollen that is carried by insects, not the wind. These rarely cause much of a problem for the child with allergies unless he or she is in very close contact with them. However, many plants have pollen that is carried by the wind, often for long distances. Because pollen can travel so far, you should be aware of plants that grow in your general area as well as those in your immediate backyard.

The air contains different amounts of pollen depending on the season and weather conditions. Pollen counts are usually lower in rainy weather. Highest counts occur in the early morning (between 4:00 and 8:00 a.m.) in warm, dry weather. Brisk winds spread pollen.

How to reduce your child's exposure to pollen

- Avoid planting many trees or shrubs near your house, especially on the side near the child's bedroom.
- Remove weeds from your garden by cutting them or using weed killers.
- Whenever possible, keep your child away from cultivated fields, construction sites, unpaved parking areas and frequently disturbed vacant lots.
- Avoid close contact with flowers both inside and outside your home. Keep cut flowers indoors to a minimum. (Dried flowers should also be limited because they collect dust and mould.)
- Do not grow plants that are related to ragweed. These include chrysanthemums, zinnias, marigolds, dahlias and sunflowers.
- Give your allergic child a bedroom on the cooler side of the house so that his or her window can be kept closed in the pollen season.
- Encourage your child to change clothes and take a bath when he or she comes indoors after playing outside in the grass. Then remove the soiled clothes until they are washed. The same rule applies to any other member of the family who is in close daily contact with plants the child is allergic to.
- Do not take long car trips in the country with the windows open.

Indoor air pollution and tobacco smoke

There are many chemicals in our homes. If odours are present and/or there isn't proper ventilation, these chemicals can affect and aggravate the allergic problem.

Outside sources of chemicals such as heavy traffic and factory smoke can be reduced by shutting windows during peak exposures. An attached garage may be a source of exhaust fumes or fumes from stored chemicals, and one should check for odours in rooms adjacent to or above a garage. Any outside vents from kitchen, bathroom and dryers should be located as high as possible so that the home is not recirculating its own exhaust fumes.

Chemicals used inside the home include such items as paints, perfumes, insecticides, hair or body sprays, cleaning agents, waxes, glues, etc. These should not be used when the child is around. If possible, keep windows open. The containers should be properly sealed and stored away from the child.

Tobacco smoke is a common indoor pollutant. It has been conclusively demonstrated that children exposed to tobacco smoke are more likely to develop throat and chest infections whether they are allergic or not. Smokers should refrain from smoking when they are near the allergic child, such as in the same room or inside a car. Having an allergic child is a good reason to stop smoking.

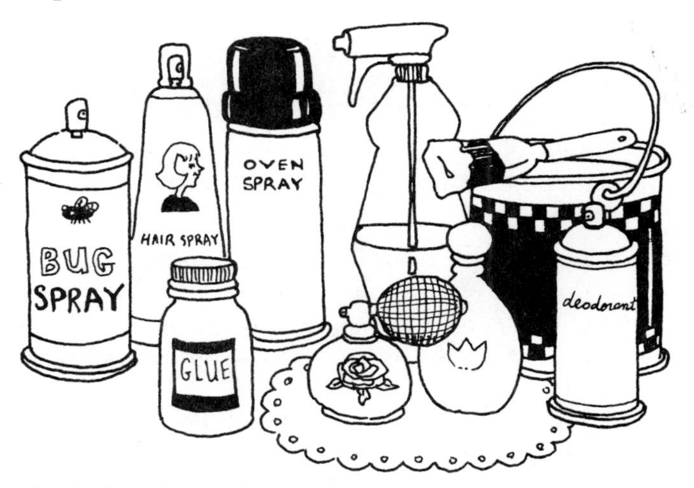

Chemicals used in the home.

Workplace irritants in the home

Some types of work involve contact with irritants. Parents or other members of the family who work with irritants should wash and change their clothes as soon as they get home from work so that they do not expose the allergic child to the irritants.

Living down wind from factories may bring irritants into your home. If possible, avoid living where the prevailing wind will carry industrial pollution (fumes, dust, etc.) into your home or yard.

Common occupational irritants

This list tells only part of the story. There are many other occupational irritants. Every year more chemicals are used in industry and new irritants appear. Here, however, are some of the more common occupational irritants.

- wood dust — mill workers and carpenters
- soldering fluxes — electricians and sheet metal workers
- cotton dust — workers in textile and vegetable oil industries
- flour and grain — bakers and farmers
- ampicillin and other drugs — pharmaceutical workers
- gases — chemical and petroleum industry workers
- metal fumes — industrial workers exposed to metallic salts.

Unusual plant allergies

Many widely used products contain plant components which can cause unusual allergies. The following three items are obvious examples.

- Pyrethrum is an insecticide made from the dried flowers of the various types of cultivated Eurasian chrysanthemum. A person who is sensitive to ragweed may react to insecticides containing pyrethrum.
- Kapok is a plant fibre used in less expensive pillows and mattresses. It is also used in boat cushions, life jackets, sleeping bags and antique furniture.

- Cottonseed is unrefined cotton. It is found along with cotton linters (short fibres from cotton seeds) in some mattresses and furniture upholstery. Cottonseed meal is used in fried cakes, fig bars, some cookies, some animal feeds and fertilizers. (Note: cottonseed oil is highly refined and does not cause problems. Refined cotton, as used in sheets, is not a problem.)

Mechanical devices for environmental control

Small changes in temperature and/or humidity can have a marked effect on your child's allergies. Very dry air, for example, when the heat is turned on, or damp areas in the home may be cause for concern. Temperature is best kept at 20 to 21 °C (68 to 70 °F) and the humidity around 35 to 50 per cent. A thermostat and a hygrometer (available in hardware stores) placed in your child's room can help you monitor and, if necessary, correct temperature and humidity.

Equipment for heating, cooling, humidifying, dehumidifying and filtering the air in your home is available but may also be expensive. These are only machines and hence cannot provide 100 per cent relief for your child, but they can help, especially if the problems are severe. Information about various kinds of equipment can be obtained from magazines such as *Canadian Consumer* and *Consumer Report*.

Some homes are now equipped with central units that help with some of the above functions. However, these may not be sufficient for your child's bedroom, especially if it is on the upper floor. Portable units may be necessary. All units, whether central or portable, require maintenance. Most have some filtering apparatus and these filters should be cleaned and/or changed more frequently than recommended by the manufacturer. As well, these units contain moisture and hence may harbour moulds which can be blown onto your child. Therefore more frequent cleaning of these units with the solutions suggested by the manufacturer is recommended.

There is no one ideal heating system for the allergic child. Forced air heating without dust filters is the least effective, as it tends to whip up the dust. To reduce the dust, filters are recommended for all individual room vents. Sealing the vents in the child's room with a layer of cheesecloth may also be helpful, provided other sources of heat such as electric blankets or baseboard heaters can be used. The furnace and duct work should be vacuumed by a professional furnace cleaning firm once a year, preferably before winter.

For cooling the home, use a central or portable air conditioning unit. Air conditioning means that windows can be closed during the summer season when pollen is worst.

Cleaning or filtration units may be helpful, but they do not remove as many pollutants as they claim to. And they do not remove particles from the air very quickly. In fact studies have not yet proven conclusively that childen's allergies benefit by using these units.

Humidifiers are helpful, especially in the winter season, if the air is very dry in the home. Units should be placed near or in the child's room. Humidifiers that shut off when the humidity is too high in the room are recommended rather than vaporizers which do not shut off. Vaporizers may overload the child with water vapour, and the size of water droplets they produce may also irritate the child. Because of this, they are best used for children who have stuffy noses and then only for short periods (i.e., a few hours on and a few hours off).

Dehumidifiers are helpful in removing excess moisture from damp areas of the house and during the summer months. This may prove helpful for the allergic child.

Although heating, cooling, air filtration, humidification and dehumidification may prove helpful for your child, the machines involved are more expensive than many of the other measures outlined in this chapter, which should be tried first.

11

Life with an allergic child: moving, travelling and visiting, school and emotions

Moving

Moving away from an area will not solve your child's allergy problems. There are no areas that are free of allergens. However, some places are worse than others. Only by living in an area will you find out how it affects your child.

A person who has allergies in one area is likely to develop allergies in another area too. The new allergies usually appear within four to six months after the move.

Travelling and visiting

Travelling may present problems for your child, but you can minimize these problems by taking certain precautions.

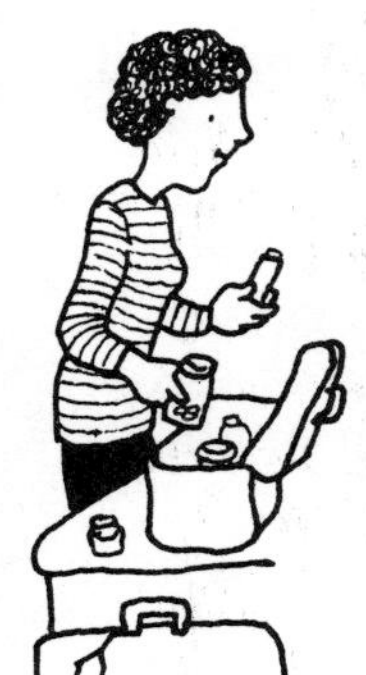

Before you leave

Always arrange your travel plans so that you are not too far from medical help in case of sudden emergencies and/or loss of medication. Make sure you have extra supplies of all essential medications. And make sure you take them with you. If you are travelling by plane, keep medications with you. Do not pack them; bags and passengers sometimes become separated.

Cars

Ensure that your car is clean and air filters are working. There should be no smoking in the car. Air conditioning is highly recommended.

Airplanes

Children with frequent ear and nose complications should take medication to help prevent pressure changes in the ear that might occur with landing and taking off. Your doctor will prescribe such medication before a trip.

Friends' homes

Instructing the parents of your child's friends about his or her problems is helpful. Dietary instructions when your child is visiting, especially if birthday celebrations are planned, can prevent problems. Sleeping over should not be a problem. You may want to send your child's pillow with him or her.

Medication

Allergy medications can be taken before visiting potential problem areas such as other homes, zoos, cottages, country areas and so on.

School

Allow your child to participate in all activities which he or she is capable of. What the child gains will more than offset any health problems caused by allergies. All children need to feel they fit in, and allergic children are no exception. Discussions with your child's teachers at the start of the school year will help to minimize problems.

If your child has frequent allergic nose or chest problems, forewarning teachers will prevent them making unnecessary requests to keep your child at home because his or her coughing and sneezing are thought to be colds.

Regardless of whether medications are to be administered by your school, the teacher should be made aware that your child is on medication. This way side effects of the drugs such as irritability, drowsiness, head or stomach pains can be reported to you.

Participation in the regular school program is essential for the child's emotional and physical well-being.

Pre-medication a half hour before a sports activity is necessary for some children, and the school should be informed of this. The child should not be pushed beyond his or her limits, but at the same time should not be made to feel inferior because of these limits. This requires a frank discussion with the physical education teacher, especially if he or she feels the child may be using allergies to get out of gym class. A letter from your doctor may be helpful in this situation.

Emotions

People used to believe that allergies were ''all in the head'' — that emotions played a large part in allergic disease. But today emotions are no longer felt to be the main culprit. Emotions can *aggravate* allergic problems, just as they can any long-term illness, but they are not the *cause*.

However, allergies and emotions may be linked in another way. The child may have feelings of inferiority or become manipulative, siblings may be jealous of the attention given to the allergic child, and parents may harbour feelings of resentment at the disruption of family life that occasionally occurs. These are all normal feelings that can be expected to surface from time to time. How you deal with them is important.

Feelings of inferiority can be overcome by allowing your child to participate in most things. Today with the medications available it is possible to pre-medicate children before sports activity or a visit to a special area. As a result, allergic children do not need to be over-protected as they were years ago.

An allergic child may try to manipulate his or her parent, siblings or friends by not taking medications or exposing him or herself to allergens that cause problems, then demanding special treatment. While it is difficult not to pamper a sick child, it is even more difficult to live with a manipulative child. Maintain discipline as you would for any other child.

Sibling jealousies can be minimized by making sure that other children in the family do not have to forfeit their rights because of a sibling's problem. Some sacrifices are inevitable. For example, a pet allergy may mean no pets even though a non-affected child desperately wants one. Such things as family outings should be planned well in advance so that the allergic child's problems can be anticipated and taken care of. Even so, a family's activities may be limited because of an allergic child. Non-affected children should have a sense that sacrifices are kept to a minimum and know the reasons why they have to be made.

Parents also need to know that it is normal at times to feel frustrated. Allergic children may demand more, but they don't demand that their parents be more perfect than anyone else.

When problems such as these arise, discuss them with your physician before the issues become intolerable. The problems you are facing are common. You and your family are not alone or unique because you have them.

Other Sources of Information

For help with your child's allergy problem or information on summer camps and organizations in your area, contact your family doctor, paediatrician or the appropriate source listed below.

Allergy Clinics and Departments in Paediatric Hospitals

If there is no paediatric hospital located near you, contact the allergy department of your local general hospital.

Allergy Clinic
Children's Hospital, Vancouver
4480 Oak St. V6H 3V4
(604) 875-2345

Allergy Clinic
Alberta Children's Provincial General Hospital, Calgary
1820 Richmond Road S.W. T2T 5C7
(403) 229-7211

Allergy Clinic
The Children's Hospital of Winnipeg, Winnipeg
c/o Health Sciences Centre
840 Sherbrook St. R3A 1M4
(204) 774-6511

Allergy Clinic
War Memorial Children's Hospital, London
c/o Victoria Hospital Corporation
375 South St. N6A 4G5
(519) 432-5241

Allergy Clinic
Children's Hospital of Eastern Ontario/
Hôpital pour enfants de l'est de l'Ontario, Ottawa
401 Smyth Rd. K1H 8L1
(613) 737-7600

Allergy Clinic
The Hospital for Sick Children, Toronto
555 University Ave. M5G 1X8
(416) 597-1500

Allergy Clinic
Hôpital Sainte-Justine, Montreal
3175 chemin Côte Ste-Catherine H3T 1C5
(514) 731-4931

Allergy Department
The Montreal Children's Hospital, Montreal
2300 Tupper St. H3H 1P3
(514) 934-4400

Allergy Clinic
Izaak Walton Killam Hospital for Children, Halifax
5850 University Ave. P.O. Box 3070 B3J 3G9
(902) 428-8111

The Dr. Charles A. Janeway Child Health Centre, St. John's
Newfoundland Dr. A1A 1R8
(709) 778-4222

Allergy Associations

The Allergy Information Association
25 Poynter Drive, Suite 7
Weston, Ont. M9R 1K8
(416) 244-9312

Allergy Foundation of Canada
Box 1904
Saskatoon, Sask. S7K 3S5
(306) 664-4618

Asthma Associations

Asthma Society of Canada
P.O. Box 213, Station K
Toronto, Ont. M4P 2G5
(416) 977-9684

Lung Associations

Parents of asthmatic children can contact their province's Lung Association (listed in the telephone book) or the Canadian Lung Association.

Canadian Lung Association
75 Albert Street, Suite 908
Ottawa, Ont. K1P 5E7
(613) 237-1208

Index